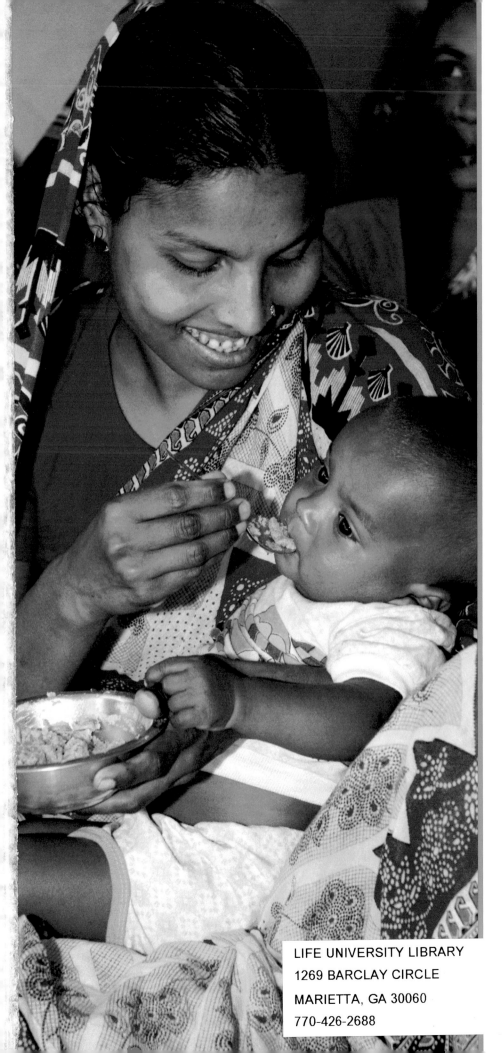

TRACKING PROGRESS ON CHILD AND MATERNAL NUTRITION

A survival and development priority

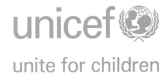

unicef

unite for children

CONTENTS

FOREWORD

Undernutrition contributes to more than one third of all deaths in children under the age of five. It does this by stealing children's strength and making illness more dangerous. An undernourished child struggles to withstand an attack of pneumonia, diarrhoea or other illness – and illness often prevails.

Undernutrition is caused by poor feeding and care, aggravated by illness. The children who survive may become locked in a cycle of recurring illness and faltering growth – diminishing their physical health, irreversibly damaging their development and their cognitive abilities, and impairing their capacities as adults. If a child suffers from diarrhoea – due to a lack of clean water or adequate sanitation, or because of poor hygiene practices – it will drain nutrients from his or her body.

And so it goes, from bad to worse: Children who are weakened by nutritional deficiencies cannot stave off illness for long, and the frequent and more severe bouts of illness they experience make them even weaker. More than a third of the children who died from pneumonia, diarrhoea and other illnesses could have survived if they had not been undernourished.

This report shows that an estimated 195 million children under age 5 in developing countries suffer from stunting, a consequence of chronic nutritional deprivation that begins in the period before birth if the mother is undernourished. Of these, more than 90 per cent are in Asia and Africa.

Maternal undernutrition affects a woman's chances of surviving pregnancy as well as her child's health. Women who were stunted as girls, whose nutritional status was poor when they conceived or who didn't gain enough weight during pregnancy may deliver babies with low birthweight. These infants in turn may never recoup from their early disadvantage. Like other undernourished children, they may be susceptible to infectious disease and death, and as adults they may face a higher risk of chronic illness such as heart disease and diabetes. Thus the health of the child is inextricably linked to the health of the mother.

In turn, the health of the mother is linked to the status a woman has in the society in which she lives. In many developing countries, the low status of women is considered to be one of the primary reasons for undernutrition across the life cycle.

Undernutrition in children under age 2 diminishes the ability of children to learn and earn throughout their lives. Nutritional deprivation leaves children tired and weak, and lowers their IQs, so they perform poorly in school. As adults they are less productive and earn less than their healthy peers. The cycle of undernutrition and poverty thereby repeats itself, generation after generation.

Exclusive breastfeeding for the first six months and continued breastfeeding together with appropriate foods can have a major impact on children's survival, growth and development. Adding vitamin A to the diet, to boost resistance to disease, and zinc, to treat diarrhoea, can further reduce child mortality. Fortification of staple foods, condiments and complementary foods for young children can make life-saving vitamins and minerals available to large segments of the population. Ensuring against iodine and iron deficiencies improves lives and cognitive development. Studies show iodine deficiency lowers IQ 13.5 points on average.

For children who suffer from severe acute malnutrition, often in the context of emergencies, ready-to-use foods can effectively reduce the malnutrition and replenish many of the nutrients and energy lost.

Lack of attention to child and maternal nutrition today will result in considerably higher costs tomorrow. With more than 1 billion people suffering from malnutrition and hunger, international leadership and urgent action are needed. Global commitments on food security, nutrition and sustainable agriculture are part of a wider international agenda that will help address the critical issues raised in this report.

Ann M. Veneman

Ann M. Veneman
Executive Director, UNICEF

GLOSSARY OF TERMS USED IN THIS REPORT

■ **Breastmilk substitute:** any food being marketed or otherwise represented as a partial or total replacement for breastmilk, whether or not it is suitable for that purpose.

■ **Complementary feeding:** the process starting when breastmilk alone or infant formula alone is no longer sufficient to meet the nutritional requirements of an infant, and therefore other foods and liquids are needed along with breastmilk or a breastmilk substitute. The target range for complementary feeding is generally considered to be 6–23 months.

■ **Exclusive breastfeeding:** infant receives only breastmilk (including breastmilk that has been expressed or from a wet nurse) and nothing else, even water or tea. Medicines, oral rehydration solution, vitamins and minerals, as recommended by health providers, are allowed during exclusive breastfeeding.

■ **Low birthweight:** an infant weighing less than 2,500 grams at birth.

■ **Malnutrition:** a broad term commonly used as an alternative to undernutrition, but technically it also refers to overnutrition. People are malnourished if their diet does not provide adequate nutrients for growth and maintenance or they are unable to fully utilize the food they eat due to illness (undernutrition). They are also malnourished if they consume too many calories (overnutrition).

■ **Micronutrients:** essential vitamins and minerals required by the body throughout the lifecycle in miniscule amounts.

■ **Micronutrient deficiency:** occurs when the body does not have sufficient amounts of a vitamin or mineral due to insufficient dietary intake and/or insufficient absorption and/or suboptimal utilization of the vitamin or mineral.

■ **Moderate acute malnutrition:** defined as weight for height between minus two and minus three standard deviations from the median weight for height of the standard reference population.

■ **Overweight:** defined as weight for height above two standard deviations from the median weight for height of the standard reference population.

■ **Stunting:** defined as height for age below minus two standard deviations from the median height for age of the standard reference population.

■ **Severe acute malnutrition:** defined as weight for height below minus three standard deviations from the median weight for height of the standard reference population, mid-upper arm circumference (MUAC) less than 115 mm, visible severe thinness, or the presence of nutritional oedema.

■ **Supplementary feeding:** additional foods provided to vulnerable groups, including moderately malnourished children.

■ **Undernutrition:** the outcome of insufficient food intake, inadequate care and infectious diseases. It includes being underweight for one's age, too short for one's age (stunting), dangerously thin for one's height (wasting) and deficient in vitamins and minerals (micronutrient deficiencies).

■ **Underweight:** a composite form of undernutrition that includes elements of stunting and wasting and is defined as weight for age below minus two standard deviations from the median weight for age of the standard reference population.

■ **Wasting:** defined as weight for height below minus two standard deviations from the median weight for height of the standard reference population. A child can be moderately wasted (between minus two and minus three standard deviations from the median weight for height) or severely wasted (below minus three standard deviations from the median weight for height).

INTRODUCTION

The first Millennium Development Goal calls for the eradication of extreme poverty and hunger, and its achievement is crucial for national progress and development.

Failing to achieve this goal jeopardizes the achievement of other MDGs, including goals to achieve universal primary education (MDG 2), reduce child mortality (MDG 4) and improve maternal health (MDG 5).

One of the indicators used to assess progress towards MDG 1 is the prevalence of children under 5 years old who are underweight, or whose weight is less than it should be for their age. To have adequate and regular weight gain, children need enough good-quality food, they need to stay healthy and they need sufficient care from their families and communities.

To a great extent, achieving the MDG target on underweight depends on the effective implementation of large-scale nutrition and health programmes that will provide appropriate food, health and care for all children in a country.

Since the MDGs were adopted in 2000, knowledge of the causes and consequences of undernutrition has greatly improved.

Recent evidence makes it clear that in children under 5 years of age, the period of greatest vulnerability to nutritional deficiencies is very early in life: the period beginning with the woman's pregnancy and continuing until the child is 2 years old. During this period, nutritional deficiencies have a significant adverse impact on child survival and growth.

Chronic undernutrition in early childhood also results in diminished cognitive and physical development, which puts children at a disadvantage for the rest of their lives. They may perform poorly in school, and as adults they may be less productive, earn less and face a higher risk of disease than adults who were not undernourished as children.

For girls, chronic undernutrition in early life, either before birth or during early childhood, can later lead to their babies being born with low birthweight, which can lead again to undernutrition as these babies grow older. Thus a vicious cycle of undernutrition repeats itself, generation after generation.

Where undernutrition is widespread, these negative consequences for individuals translate into negative consequences for countries. Knowing whether children are at risk of nutritional deficiencies, and taking appropriate actions to prevent and treat such deficiencies, is therefore imperative.

Whether a child has experienced chronic nutritional deficiencies and frequent bouts of illness in early life is best indicated by the infant's growth in length and the child's growth in height. Day-to-day nutritional deficiencies over a period of time lead to diminished, or stunted, growth. Once children are stunted, it is difficult for them to catch up in height later on, especially if they are living in conditions that prevail in many developing countries.

Whereas a deficit in height (stunting) is difficult to correct, a deficit in weight (underweight) can be recouped if nutrition and health improve later in childhood. The weight of a child at 4–5 years old, when it is adequate for the child's age, can therefore mask deficiencies that occurred during pregnancy or infancy, and growth and development that have been compromised.

The global burden of stunting is far greater than the burden of underweight. This report, which is based on the latest available data, shows that in the developing world the number of children under 5 years old who are stunted is close to 200 million, while the number of children under 5 who are underweight is about 130 million. Indeed, many countries have much higher rates of stunting prevalence among children compared with underweight prevalence.

Governments, donors and partners that consider only underweight prevalence are overlooking a significant portion of the persistent problem of undernutrition. The high stunting burden in many countries should be an issue of great concern, as pointed out in this report.

Today, there is a much better understanding of the programme strategies and approaches to improve nutrition, based on sound evidence and improved health and nutrition data. This report draws on these sources in order to identify key factors for the effective implementation of programmes to improve maternal nutrition, breastfeeding, complementary feeding, and vitamin and mineral intake for infants and young children. The report also provides information that demonstrates that improving child nutrition is entirely feasible.

It describes, for example, how cost-effective nutrition interventions such as vitamin A supplementation reach the vast majority of children even in the least developed countries; that great progress has been made to improve infant feeding in many African countries; and that the treatment of severe acute malnutrition has expanded rapidly.

The large burden of undernutrition, and its influence on poverty reduction as well as the achievement of many of the MDGs, itself constitutes a call for action. The fact that even more children may become undernourished in some countries due to such recent events as the rapid increase in food prices and the financial crisis brings acute focus to the issue.

Given what is now known about the serious, long-lasting impact of undernutrition, as well as about experiences of effective and innovative programme approaches to promoting good nutrition, this report is particularly timely. Its value lies in that it argues for nutrition as a core pillar of human development and in that it documents how concrete, large-scale programming not only can reduce the burden of undernutrition and deprivation in countries but also can advance the progress of nations.

KEY MESSAGES

Overview

- Undernutrition jeopardizes children's survival, health, growth and development, and it slows national progress towards development goals. Undernutrition is often an invisible problem.

- A child's future nutrition status is affected before conception and is greatly dependent on the mother's nutrition status prior to and during pregnancy. A chronically undernourished woman will give birth to a baby who is likely to be undernourished as a child, causing the cycle of undernutrition to be repeated over generations.

- Children with iron and iodine deficiencies do not perform as well in school as their well-nourished peers, and when they grow up they may be less productive than other adults.

- Stunting reflects chronic nutritional deficiency, aggravated by illness. Compared to other forms of undernutrition, it is a problem of larger proportions:
  - Among children under 5 years old in the developing world, an estimated one third – 195 million children – are stunted, whereas 129 million are underweight.
  - Twenty-four countries bear 80 per cent of the developing world burden of undernutrition as measured by stunting.
  - In Africa and Asia, stunting rates are particularly high, at 40 per cent and 36 per cent respectively. More than 90 per cent of the developing world's stunted children live in Africa and Asia.

- Progress for children lies at the heart of all Millennium Development Goals (MDGs). Along with cognitive and physical development, proper nutrition contributes significantly to declines in under-five mortality rates, reductions of disease and poverty, improvements in maternal health and gender equality – thus, it is essential for achieving most of the MDGs.

Programme evidence

- There is a critical window of opportunity to prevent undernutrition – while a mother is pregnant and during a child's first two years of life – when proven nutrition interventions offer children the best chance to survive and reach optimal growth and development.

- Marked reductions in child undernutrition can be achieved through improvements in women's nutrition before and during pregnancy, early and exclusive breastfeeding, and good-quality complementary feeding for infants and young children, with appropriate micronutrient interventions.

- Large-scale programmes – including the promotion, protection and support of exclusive breastfeeding, providing vitamins and minerals through fortified foods and supplements, and community-based treatment of severe acute malnutrition – have been successful in many countries. Where such programming does not yet exist, this experience can guide implementation at scale.

- Unsafe water, inadequate sanitation and poor hygiene increase the risk of diarrhoea and other illnesses that deplete children of vital nutrients and can lead to chronic undernutrition and increase the risk of death.

- Improving child and maternal nutrition is not only entirely feasible but also affordable and cost-effective. Nutrition interventions are among the best investments in development that countries can undertake.

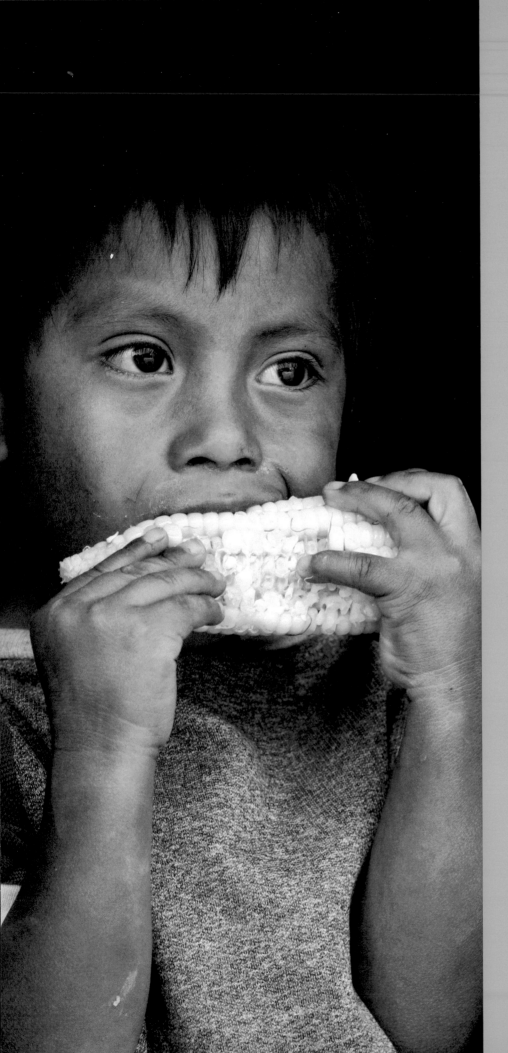

OVERVIEW

1. THE CHALLENGE OF UNDERNUTRITION

The level of child and maternal undernutrition remains unacceptable throughout the world, with 90 per cent of the developing world's chronically undernourished (stunted) children living in Asia and Africa. Detrimental and often undetected until severe, undernutrition undermines the survival, growth and development of children and women, and it diminishes the strength and capacity of nations.

Brought about by a combined lack of quality food, frequent attacks of infectious disease and deficient care, undernutrition continues to be widely prevalent in both developing and industrialized countries, to different degrees and in different forms. Nutritional deficiencies are particularly harmful while a woman is pregnant and during a child's first two years of life. During this period, they pose a significant threat to mothers and to children's survival, growth and development, which in turn negatively affects children's ability to learn in school, and to work and prosper as adults.

Undernutrition greatly impedes countries' socio-economic development and potential to reduce poverty. Many of the Millennium Development Goals (MDGs) – particularly MDG 1 (eradicate extreme poverty and hunger), MDG 4 (reduce child mortality) and MDG 5 (improve maternal health) – will not be reached unless the nutrition of

80 per cent of the developing world's stunted children live in 24 countries

24 countries with the largest numbers of children under 5 years old who are moderately or severely stunted

Ranking	Country	Stunting prevalence (%)	Number of children who are stunted (thousands, 2008)	Percentage of developing world total (195.1 million)
1	India	48	60,788	31.2%
2	China	15	12,685	6.5%
3	Nigeria	41	10,158	5.2%
4	Pakistan	42	9,868	5.1%
5	Indonesia	37	7,688	3.9%
6	Bangladesh	43	7,219	3.7%
7	Ethiopia	51	6,768	3.5%
8	Democratic Republic of the Congo	46	5,382	2.8%
9	Philippines	34	3,617	1.9%
10	United Republic of Tanzania	44	3,359	1.7%
11	Afghanistan	59	2,910	1.5%
12	Egypt	29	2,730	1.4%
13	Viet Nam	36	2,619	1.3%
14	Uganda	38	2,355	1.2%
15	Sudan	40	2,305	1.2%
16	Kenya	35	2,269	1.2%
17	Yemen	58	2,154	1.1%
18	Myanmar	41	1,880	1.0%
19	Nepal	49	1,743	<1%
20	Mozambique	44	1,670	<1%
21	Madagascar	53	1,622	<1%
22	Mexico	16	1,594	<1%
23	Niger	47	1,473	<1%
24	South Africa	27	1,425	<1%
				Total: 80%

Note: Estimates are based on the 2006 WHO Child Growth Standards, except for the following countries where estimates are available only according to the previous NCHS/WHO reference population: Kenya, Mozambique, South Africa and Viet Nam. All prevalence data based on surveys conducted in 2003 or later with the exception of Pakistan (2001–2002). For more information on the prevalence and number estimates, see the data notes on page 116.

Source: Multiple Indicator Cluster Surveys (MICS), Demographic and Health Surveys (DHS) and other national surveys, 2003–2008.

women and children is prioritized in national development programmes and strategies. With persistently high levels of undernutrition in the developing world, vital opportunities to save millions of lives are being lost, and many more children are not growing and thriving to their full potential.

In terms of numbers, the bulk of the world's undernutrition problem is localized. Twenty-four countries account for more than 80 per cent of the global burden of chronic undernutrition, as measured by stunting (low height for age). Although India does not have the highest prevalence of stunted children, due to its large population it has the greatest number of stunted children.

Stunting remains a problem of greater magnitude than underweight or wasting, and it more accurately reflects nutritional deficiencies and illness that occur during the most critical periods for growth and development in early life. Most countries have stunting rates that are much higher than their underweight rates, and in some countries, more than half of children under 5 years old are stunted.

Nutrition remains a low priority on the national development agendas of many countries, despite clear evidence of the consequences of nutritional deprivation in the short and long term. The reasons are multiple.

Nutrition problems are often unnoticed until they reach a severe level. But mild and moderate undernutrition are highly prevalent and carry consequences of enormous magnitude: growth impediment, impaired learning ability and, later in life, low work productivity. None of these conditions is as visible as the diseases from which the undernourished child dies. Children may appear to be healthy even when they face grave risks associated with undernutrition. Not recognizing the urgency, policymakers may not understand how improved nutrition relates to national economic and social goals.

18 countries with the highest prevalence of stunting

Prevalence of moderate and severe stunting among children under 5 years old, in 18 countries where the prevalence rate is 45 per cent or more

Country	Prevalence of stunting (moderate and severe) (%)
Afghanistan	59
Yemen	58
Guatemala	54
Timor-Leste	54
Burundi	53
Madagascar	53
Malawi	53
Ethiopia	51
Rwanda	51
Nepal	49
Bhutan	48
India	48
Lao People's Democratic Republic	48
Guinea-Bissau	47
Niger	47
Democratic Republic of the Congo	46
Democratic People's Republic of Korea	45
Zambia	45

Note: Estimates are calculated according to the WHO Child Growth Standards, except in cases where data are only available according to the previously used NCHS/WHO reference population; please refer to data notes on page 116 for more information. Estimates are based on data collection in 2003 or later, with the exception of Guatemala (2002) and Bhutan (1999).

Source: MICS, DHS and other national surveys, 2003–2008.

In many countries, nutrition has no clear institutional home; it is often addressed in part by various ministries or departments, an arrangement that can hinder effective planning and management of programmes.

In some of the countries with the highest levels of undernutrition, governments are faced with multiple challenges – poverty, economic crisis, conflict, disaster, inequity – all of them urgent, and all of them competing for attention. Undernutrition often does not feature prominently among these problems, unless it becomes very severe and widespread.

Some leaders may not consider nutrition to be politically expedient because it requires investment over the long term and the results are not always immediately visible. Furthermore, the interests of donor agencies – with limited budgetary allocations for aid in general – are often focused elsewhere.

In the past, nutrition strategies were not always effective and comprehensive, programmes were insufficient in scale and human resources were woefully inadequate, partly due to insufficient coordination and collaboration between international institutions and agencies working in nutrition. But cost-effective programming strategies and interventions that can make a significant difference in the health and lives of children and women are available today. These interventions urgently require scaling up, a task that will entail the collective planning and resources of developing country governments at all levels and of the international development community as a whole.

Undernutrition can be greatly reduced through the delivery of simple interventions at key stages of the life cycle – for the mother, before she becomes pregnant, during pregnancy and while breastfeeding; for the child, in infancy and early childhood. Effectively scaled up, these interventions will improve maternal nutrition, increase the proportion of infants who are exclusively breastfed up to 6 months of age, improve continued breastfeeding rates, enhance complementary feeding and micronutrient intake of children between 6 and 24 months old, and reduce the severity of infectious diseases and child mortality.

Undernutrition is a violation of child rights. The Convention on the Rights of the Child emphasizes children's right to the highest attainable standard of health and places responsibility on the State to combat malnutrition. It also requires that nutritious food is provided to children and that all segments of society are supported in the use of basic knowledge of child nutrition (article 24). Nutrition must be placed high on national and international agendas if this right is to be fulfilled.

2. THE IMPORTANCE OF NUTRITION

Consequences of undernutrition and the impact of nutrition interventions on child survival

Children who are undernourished, not optimally breastfed or suffering from micronutrient deficiencies have substantially lower chances of survival than children who are well nourished. They are much more likely to suffer from a serious infection and to die from common childhood illnesses such as diarrhoea, measles, pneumonia and malaria, as well as HIV and AIDS.[1]

According to the most recent estimates, maternal and child undernutrition contributes to more than one third of child deaths.[2] Undernourished children who survive may become locked in a cycle of recurring illness and faltering growth, with irreversible damage to their development and cognitive abilities.[3]

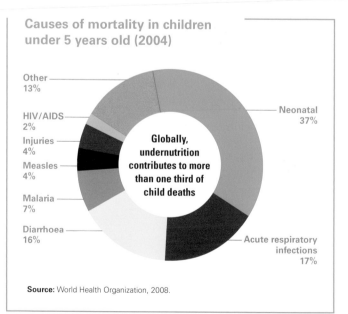

Causes of mortality in children under 5 years old (2004)

Globally, undernutrition contributes to more than one third of child deaths

- Other 13%
- HIV/AIDS 2%
- Injuries 4%
- Measles 4%
- Malaria 7%
- Diarrhoea 16%
- Neonatal 37%
- Acute respiratory infections 17%

Source: World Health Organization, 2008.

Every level of undernutrition increases the risk of a child's dying. While children suffering from severe acute malnutrition are more than nine times more likely to die than children who are not undernourished,[4] a large number of deaths also occurs among moderately and mildly undernourished children who may otherwise appear healthy. Compared to children who are severely undernourished, children who are moderately or mildly undernourished have a lower risk of dying, but there are many more of the latter.[5]

Manifestations of inadequate nutrition

Undernutrition in children can manifest itself in several ways, and it is most commonly assessed through the measurement of weight and height. A child can be too short for his or her age (stunted), have low weight for his or her height (wasted), or have low weight for his or her age (underweight). A child who is underweight can also be stunted or wasted or both.

Each of these indicators captures a certain aspect of the problem. Weight is known to be a sensitive indicator of acute deficiencies, whereas height captures more chronic exposure to deficiencies and infections. Wasting is used as a way to identify severe acute malnutrition.

Inadequate nutrition may also manifest itself in overweight and obesity, commonly assessed through the body mass index.

Micronutrient malnutrition, caused by deficiencies in vitamins and minerals, can manifest itself through such conditions as fatigue, pallor associated with anaemia (iron deficiency), reduced learning ability (mainly iron and iodine deficiency), goitre (iodine deficiency), reduced immunity, and night blindness (severe vitamin A deficiency).

Low birthweight is related to maternal undernutrition; it contributes to infections and asphyxia, which together account for 60 per cent of neonatal deaths. An infant born weighing between 1,500 and 2,000 grams is eight times more likely to die than an infant born with an adequate weight of at least 2,500 grams. Low birthweight causes an estimated 3.3 per cent of overall child deaths.[6]

Thus, the achievement of Millennium Development Goal 4 – to reduce the under-five mortality rate by two thirds between 1990 and 2015 – will not be possible without urgent, accelerated and concerted action to improve maternal and child nutrition.

Food and nutrition

Undernutrition is not just about the lack of food. An individual's nutritional status is influenced by three broad categories of factors – food, care and health – and adequate nutrition requires the presence of all three.

Poor infant and young child feeding and care, along with illnesses such as diarrhoea, pneumonia, malaria, and HIV and AIDS, often exacerbated by intestinal parasites, are immediate causes of undernutrition. Underlying and more basic causes include poverty, illiteracy, social norms and behaviour.

Maternal nutrition and health greatly influence child nutritional status. A woman's low weight for height or anaemia during pregnancy can lead to low birthweight and continued undernutrition in her children. At the same time, maternal undernutrition increases the risk of maternal death during childbirth.

Household food security, often influenced by such factors as poverty, drought and other emergencies, has an important role in determining the state of child and maternal nutrition in many countries.

Optimal infant and young child feeding – initiation of breastfeeding within one hour of birth, exclusive breastfeeding for the first six months of the child's life and continued breastfeeding until the child is at least 2 years old, together with age-appropriate, nutritionally adequate and safe complementary foods – can have a major impact on child survival, with the potential to prevent an estimated 19 per cent of all under-5 deaths in the developing world, more than any other preventive intervention.[7] In the conditions that normally exist in developing countries, breastfed children are at least 6 times more likely to survive in the early months than non-breastfed children; in the first six months of life they are 6 times less likely to die from diarrhoea and 2.4 times less likely to die from acute respiratory infection.[8]

Vitamin A is critical for the body's immune system; supplementation of this micronutrient can reduce the risk of child mortality from all causes by about 23 per cent. The provision of high-dose vitamin A supplements twice a year to all children 6–59 months old in countries with high child mortality rates is one of the most cost-effective interventions.[9] Zinc supplementation can reduce the prevalence of diarrhoea in children by 27 per cent because it shortens the duration and reduces the severity of a diarrhoea episode.[10]

Consequences of undernutrition and the impact of nutrition interventions on development, school performance and income

The period of children's most rapid physical growth and development is also the period of their greatest vulnerability. Significant brain formation and development takes place beginning from the time the child is in the womb. Adequate nutrition – providing the right amount of carbohydrates, protein, fats, and vitamins and minerals – is essential during the antenatal and early childhood period.

Maternal undernutrition, particularly low body mass index, which can cause fetal growth retardation, and non-optimal infant and young child feeding are the main causes of faltering growth and undernutrition in children under 2 years old.[11] These conditions can have a lifelong negative impact on brain structure and function.

Stunting is an important predictor of child development; it is associated with reduced school outcome. Compared to children who are not stunted, stunted children often enrol later, complete fewer grades and perform less well in school. In turn, this underperformance leads to reduced productivity and income-earning capacity in adult life.[12]

Iodine and iron deficiency can also undermine children's school performance. Studies show that children from communities that are iodine deficient can lose 13.5 IQ points on average compared with children from communities that are non-deficient,[13] and the intelligence quotients of children suffering iron deficiency in early infancy were lower than those of their peers who were not deficient.[14] Iron deficiency makes children tired, slow and listless, so they do not perform well in school.

Iron-deficiency anaemia is highly prevalent among women in developing-country settings and increases the risk of maternal death.[15] It causes weakness and fatigue, and reduces their physical ability to work. Adults suffering from anaemia are reported to be less productive than adults who are not anaemic.[16]

Early childhood is also a critical period for a child's cognitive development. Particularly in settings where ill health and undernutrition are common, it is important to stimulate the child's cognitive development during the first two years through interaction and play. Nutrition and child development interventions have a synergistic effect on growth and development outcomes.

Nutrition in early childhood has a lasting impact on health and well-being in adulthood. Children with deficient growth before age 2 are at an increased risk of chronic disease as adults if they gain weight rapidly in later stages of childhood.[17] For chronic conditions such as cardiovascular disease and diabetes, a worst-case scenario is a baby of low birthweight who is stunted and underweight in infancy and then gains weight rapidly in childhood and adult life.[18] This scenario is not uncommon in countries where underweight rates have been reduced but stunting remains relatively high.

Undernutrition has dominated discussions on nutritional status in developing countries, but overweight among both children and adults has emerged in many countries as a public health issue, especially in countries undergoing a so-called 'nutrition transition'. Overweight is caused in these countries mainly by poverty and by poor infant and young child feeding practices; the 'transition' refers to changes in traditional diets, with increased consumption of high-calorie, high-fat and processed foods.

Height at 2 years of age is clearly associated with enhanced productivity and human capital in adulthood,[19] so early nutrition is also an important contributor to economic development. There is evidence that improving growth through adequate complementary feeding can have a significant effect on adult wages. An evaluation of one programme in Latin America that provided good-quality complementary food to infant and young boys found their wages in adulthood increased by 46 per cent compared to peers who did not participate in the programme.[20]

3. CURRENT STATUS OF NUTRITION

Stunting

Stunting affects approximately 195 million children under 5 years old in the developing world, or about one in three. Africa and Asia have high stunting rates – 40 per cent and 36 per cent, respectively – and more than 90 per cent of the world's stunted children live on these two continents.

Of the 10 countries that contribute most to the global burden of stunting among children, 6 are in Asia. These countries all have relatively large populations: Bangladesh, China, India, Indonesia, Pakistan and the Philippines.

Due to the high prevalence of stunting (48 per cent) in combination with a large population, India alone has an estimated 61 million stunted children, accounting for more than 3 out of every 10 stunted children in the developing world.

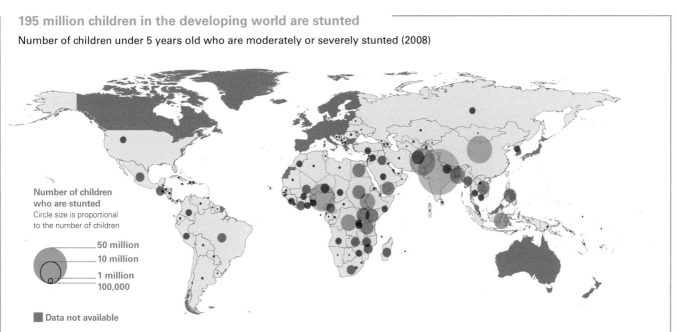

195 million children in the developing world are stunted

Number of children under 5 years old who are moderately or severely stunted (2008)

Number of children who are stunted
Circle size is proportional to the number of children

- 50 million
- 10 million
- 1 million
- 100,000

Data not available

Stunting prevalence worldwide

Percentage of children under 5 years old who are moderately or severely stunted

- Less than 5 per cent
- 5–19 per cent
- 20–29 per cent
- 30–39 per cent
- 40 per cent or more
- Data not available

Notes for all maps in this publication: The maps in this publication are stylized and not to scale. They do not reflect a position by UNICEF on the legal status of any country or territory or the delimitation of any frontiers. The dotted line represents approximately the Line of Control in Jammu and Kashmir agreed upon by India and Pakistan. The final status of Jammu and Kashmir has not yet been agreed upon by the parties. For detailed notes on the map data, see page 42.

Sources for both maps on this page: MICS, DHS and other national surveys, 2003–2008.

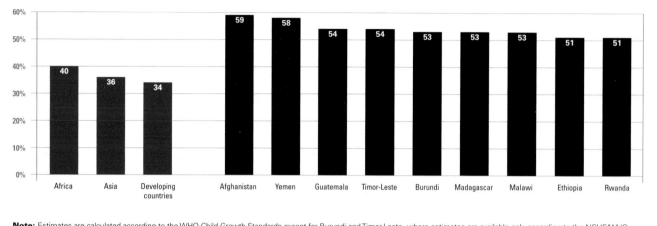

Stunting prevalence in Africa and Asia and in countries where more than half of children are stunted

Percentage of children under 5 years old who are moderately or severely stunted (based on WHO Child Growth Standards)

Africa	40
Asia	36
Developing countries	34
Afghanistan	59
Yemen	58
Guatemala	54
Timor-Leste	54
Burundi	53
Madagascar	53
Malawi	53
Ethiopia	51
Rwanda	51

Note: Estimates are calculated according to the WHO Child Growth Standards except for Burundi and Timor-Leste, where estimates are available only according to the NCHS/WHO reference population. Estimates are based on data collected in 2003 or later with the exception of Guatemala (2002).

Source: MICS, DHS and other national surveys, 2003–2008.

More than half the children under 5 years old are stunted in nine countries, including Guatemala, whose stunting rate of 54 per cent rivals that of some of the highest-prevalence countries in Africa and Asia. Of countries with available data, Afghanistan and Yemen have the highest stunting rates: 59 per cent and 58 per cent, respectively.

A nation's average rate of stunting may mask disparities. For example, an analysis of disparities in Honduras indicates that children living in the poorest households or whose mothers are uneducated have almost a 50 per cent chance of being stunted, whereas on average, throughout the country 29 per cent of children are stunted.[21]

Reducing stunting in Peru

The stunting rate in Peru is high, particularly among those who are poor. One reason for the continued high prevalence of stunting is the perception that undernutrition is primarily a food security issue. But in some regions of the country, more holistic, community-based efforts to improve basic health practices have led to an improvement in stunting levels among young children.

In 1999, the programme 'A Good Start in Life' was initiated in five regions – four in the Andean highlands and one in the Amazon region – as a collaboration between the Ministry of Health, the United States Agency for International Development and UNICEF. Efforts focused on reaching pregnant and lactating women. Methods included such community-based interventions as antenatal care, promotion of adequate food intake during pregnancy and lactation, promotion of exclusive breastfeeding of infants under 6 months of age and improved complementary feeding from six months, growth promotion, control of iron and vitamin A deficiency, promotion of iodized salt, and personal and family hygiene.

Programme teams were led by local governments, which worked with communities, health facility staff and local non-governmental organizations. The programme emphasized strengthening the capacity and skills of female counsellors and rural health promoters. By 2004, it covered the inhabitants of 223 poor, rural communities, including approximately 75,000 children under 3 years old, and 35,000 pregnant and lactating women.

A comparison between 2000 and 2004 shows that in the communities covered by the programme the stunting rate for children under 3 years old declined from 54 per cent to 37 per cent, while anaemia rates dropped from 76 per cent to 52 per cent. The total cost of the programme was estimated to be US$116.50 per child per year. 'A Good Start in Life' inspired the design and implementation of a national programme, which has since been associated with reduced stunting rates.

Source: Lechtig, Aaron, et al., 'Decreasing Stunting, Anemia, and Vitamin A Deficiency in Peru: Results of the Good Start in Life Program', *Food and Nutrition Bulletin*, vol. 30, no. 1, March 2009, pp. 37–48; and UNICEF Peru Country Office, 'Annual Report 2000' (internal document).

Decline in stunting prevalence in Africa and Asia and in countries where prevalence has decreased by more than 20 percentage points

Percentage of children under 5 years old who are moderately or severely stunted (based on NCHS/WHO reference population)

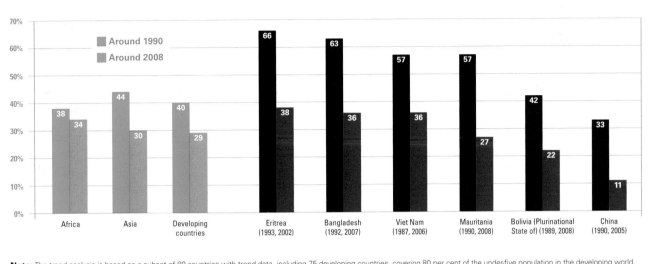

Note: The trend analysis is based on a subset of 80 countries with trend data, including 75 developing countries, covering 80 per cent of the under-five population in the developing world. All trend estimates are calculated according to the NCHS/WHO reference population.

Source: MICS, DHS and other national surveys, around 1990 to around 2008.

Since 1990, stunting prevalence in the developing world has declined from 40 per cent to 29 per cent, a relative reduction of 28 per cent. Progress has been particularly notable in Asia, where prevalence dropped from 44 per cent around 1990 to 30 per cent around 2008. This reduction is influenced by marked declines in China.

The decline in Africa has been modest, from 38 per cent around 1990 to 34 per cent around 2008. Moreover, due to population growth, the overall number of African children under 5 years old who are stunted has increased, from an estimated 43 million in 1990 to 52 million in 2008.

Stunting rates have declined significantly in a number of countries – including Bangladesh, Eritrea, Mauritania and Viet Nam – underscoring that marked improvements can be achieved. In countries where the burden of stunting is high, there is an urgent need to accelerate integrated programmes addressing nutrition during the mother's pregnancy and before the child reaches 2 years of age.

Underweight

Today, an estimated 129 million children under 5 years old in the developing world are underweight – nearly one in four. Ten per cent of children in the developing world are severely underweight. The prevalence of underweight among children is higher in Asia than in Africa, with rates of 27 per cent and 21 per cent, respectively.

Underweight prevalence in Africa and Asia and in countries where more than one third of children are underweight

Percentage of children under 5 years old who are moderately or severely underweight (based on WHO Child Growth Standards)

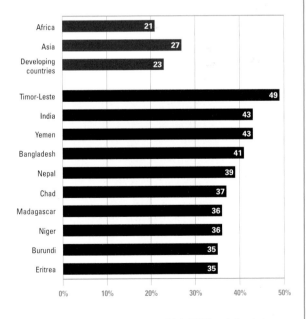

Note: Estimates are calculated according to the WHO Child Growth Standards except for Chad and Timor-Leste, where estimates are available only according to the NCHS/WHO reference population. Estimates are based on data collected in 2003 or later with the exception of Eritrea (2002).

Source: MICS, DHS and other national surveys, 2003–2008.

Underweight prevalence worldwide

Percentage of children under 5 years old who are moderately or severely underweight

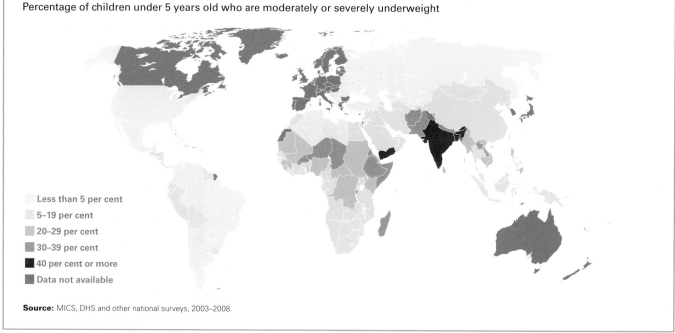

Less than 5 per cent
5–19 per cent
20–29 per cent
30–39 per cent
40 per cent or more
Data not available

Source: MICS, DHS and other national surveys, 2003–2008.

In 17 countries, underweight prevalence among children under 5 years old is greater than 30 per cent. The rates are highest in Bangladesh, India, Timor-Leste and Yemen, with more than 40 per cent of children underweight.

Contribution to the underweight burden

Countries with the largest numbers of children under five who are moderately or severely underweight, as a proportion of the developing world total (129 million children)

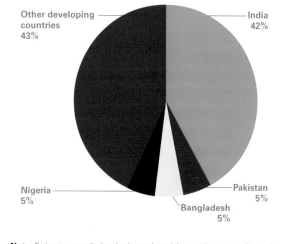

Other developing countries 43%

India 42%

Nigeria 5%

Bangladesh 5%

Pakistan 5%

Note: Estimates are calculated using underweight prevalence according to the WHO Child Growth Standards and the number of children under 5 years old in 2008. Underweight prevalence estimates are based on data collected in 2003 or later with the exception of Pakistan (2001–2002).

Source: MICS, DHS and other national surveys, 2003–2008.

Some countries have low underweight prevalence but unacceptably high stunting rates. For example, in Albania, Egypt, Iraq, Mongolia, Peru and Swaziland, stunting rates are more than 25 per cent although underweight prevalence is 6 per cent or less. For national development and public health, it is important to reduce both stunting and underweight.

Progress towards the reduction of underweight prevalence has been limited in Africa, with 28 per cent of children under 5 years old being underweight around 1990, compared with 25 per cent around 2008. Progress has been slightly better in Asia, with 37 per cent underweight prevalence around 1990 and 31 per cent around 2008.

Even in countries where underweight prevalence is low, stunting rates can be alarmingly high

Countries with underweight prevalence of 6 per cent or less and stunting rates of more than 25 per cent

Country	Prevalence of underweight (%)	Prevalence of stunting (%)	Ratio of stunting to underweight
Peru	6	30	5.4
Mongolia	5	27	5.4
Swaziland	5	29	5.4
Egypt	6	29	4.8
Albania	6	26	4.3
Iraq	6	26	4.3

Note: Estimates are calculated according to WHO Child Growth Standards.

Source: MICS, DHS and other national surveys, 2003–2008.

Decline in underweight prevalence in Africa and Asia and in the five countries with the greatest reductions

Percentage of children under 5 years old who are moderately or severely underweight (based on NCHS/WHO reference population)

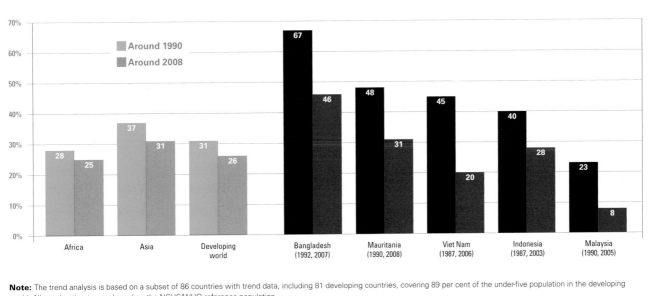

Legend:
- Around 1990
- Around 2008

Category	Around 1990	Around 2008
Africa	28	25
Asia	37	31
Developing world	31	26
Bangladesh (1992, 2007)	67	46
Mauritania (1990, 2008)	48	31
Viet Nam (1987, 2006)	45	20
Indonesia (1987, 2003)	40	28
Malaysia (1990, 2005)	23	8

Note: The trend analysis is based on a subset of 86 countries with trend data, including 81 developing countries, covering 89 per cent of the under-five population in the developing world. All trend estimates are based on the NCHS/WHO reference population.

Source: MICS, DHS and other national surveys, around 1990 to around 2008.

Sixty-three countries (out of 117 with available data) are on track to achieving the MDG 1 target of a 50 per cent reduction of underweight prevalence among children under 5 between 1990 and 2015. This compares with 46 countries (out of 94 with available data) on track just three years ago, based on trend data from around 1990 to around 2004. Today, in 34 countries, progress is insufficient, and 20 have made no progress towards achieving the MDG target. Most of these 20 countries are in Africa.

63 countries are on track to meet the MDG 1 target

Progress is insufficient to meet the MDG target in 34 countries, and 20 countries have made no progress

- **On track:** Average annual rate of reduction (AARR) in underweight prevalence is greater than or equal to 2.6 per cent, or latest available estimate of underweight prevalence estimate is less than or equal to 5 per cent, regardless of AARR
- **Insufficient progress:** AARR is between 0.6 per cent and 2.5 per cent
- **No progress:** AARR is less than or equal to 0.5 per cent
- Data not available

Source: MICS, DHS and other national surveys, around 1990 to around 2008.

Wasting

Children who suffer from wasting face a markedly increased risk of death. According to the latest available data, 13 per cent of children under 5 years old in the developing world are wasted, and 5 per cent are severely wasted (an estimated 26 million children).

A number of African and Asian countries have wasting rates that exceed 15 per cent, including Bangladesh (17 per cent), India (20 per cent) and the Sudan (16 per cent). The country with the highest prevalence of wasting in the world is Timor-Leste, where 25 per cent of children under 5 years old are wasted (8 per cent severely).

Out of 134 countries with available data, 32 have wasting prevalence of 10 per cent or more among children under 5 years old. At such elevated levels, wasting is considered a public health emergency requiring immediate intervention, in the form of emergency feeding programmes.

Ten countries account for 60 per cent of children in the developing world who suffer from wasting. The top eight countries all have wasting prevalence of 10 per cent or higher. More than one third of the developing world's children who are wasted live in India.

The burden of severe wasting is particularly high – 6 per cent or more – in countries with large populations; Indonesia, Nigeria, Pakistan and the Sudan, in addition to India, all have high rates of wasting.

10 countries account for 60 per cent of the global wasting burden

10 countries with the largest numbers of children under 5 years old who are wasted

| Country | Wasting | | | |
| | Moderate and severe | | Severe | |
	Numbers (thousands)	Prevalence (%)	Numbers (thousands)	Prevalence (%)
India	25,075	20	8,105	6
Nigeria	3,478	14	1,751	7
Pakistan	3,376	14	1,403	6
Bangladesh	2,908	17	485	3
Indonesia	2,841	14	1,295	6
Ethiopia	1,625	12	573	4
Democratic Republic of the Congo	1,183	10	509	4
Sudan	945	16	403	7
Egypt	680	7	302	3
Philippines	642	6	171	2

Note: Estimates are calculated according to the WHO Child Growth Standards, except in cases where data are only available according to the previously used NCHS/WHO reference population. For more information, please refer to data notes on page 116. China is not included due to lack of data.

Source: MICS, DHS and other national surveys, 2003–2008.

Overweight

Although being overweight is a problem most often associated with industrialized countries, some developing countries and countries in transition also have high prevalence of overweight children. In Georgia, Guinea-Bissau, Iraq, Kazakhstan, Sao Tome and Principe, and the Syrian Arab Republic, for example, 15 per cent or more of children under 5 years old are overweight.

Some countries are experiencing a 'double burden' of malnutrition, having high rates of both stunting and overweight. In Guinea-Bissau and Malawi, for example, more than 10 per cent of children are overweight, while around half are stunted.

Wasting prevalence

Percentage of children under 5 years old who are moderately or severely wasted

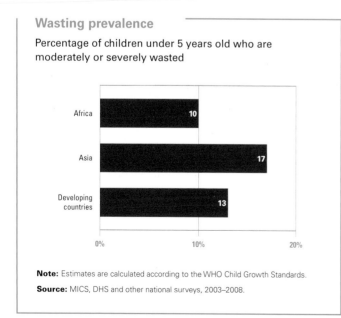

Note: Estimates are calculated according to the WHO Child Growth Standards.

Source: MICS, DHS and other national surveys, 2003–2008.

Wasting prevalence

Percentage of children under 5 years old who are moderately or severely wasted

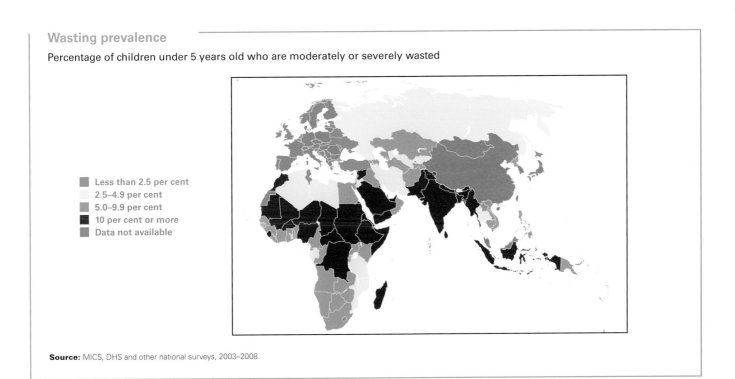

Less than 2.5 per cent
2.5–4.9 per cent
5.0–9.9 per cent
10 per cent or more
Data not available

Source: MICS, DHS and other national surveys, 2003–2008.

More than 10 per cent of children are overweight in 17 countries with available data

Percentage of children under 5 years old who are overweight and percentage who are stunted

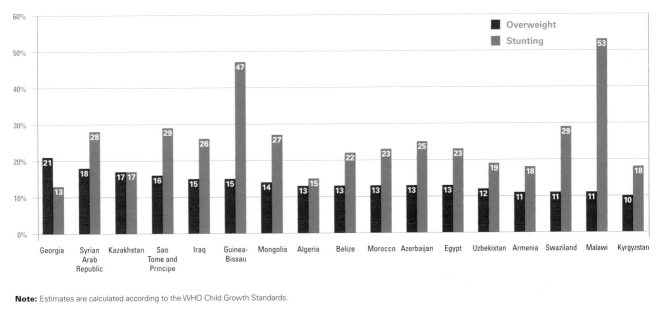

Note: Estimates are calculated according to the WHO Child Growth Standards.

Source: MICS, DHS and other national surveys, 2003–2008.

Low birthweight

In developing countries, 16 per cent of infants, or 1 in 6, weigh less than 2,500 grams at birth. Asia has the highest incidence of low birthweight by far, with 18 per cent of all infants weighing less than 2,500 grams at birth. Mauritania, Pakistan, the Sudan and Yemen all have an estimated low birthweight incidence of more than 30 per cent.

A total of 19 million newborns per year in the developing world are born with low birthweight, and India has the highest number of low birthweight babies per year: 7.4 million.

The low proportion of newborns who are weighed at birth indicates a lack of appropriate newborn care and may lead to inaccurate estimates of low-birthweight incidence. Almost 60 per cent of newborns in developing countries are not weighed at birth. Some countries with very high incidence of low birthweight also have a very high rate of infants who are not weighed at birth. In Pakistan and Yemen, for example, where almost one third of newborns are estimated to be of low birthweight, more than 90 per cent of infants are not weighed at birth.

Contribution to the low birthweight burden

Countries with the largest numbers of infants weighing less than 2,500 grams at birth, as a proportion of the global total (19 million newborns per year)

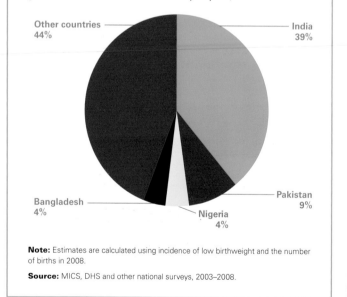

Note: Estimates are calculated using incidence of low birthweight and the number of births in 2008.

Source: MICS, DHS and other national surveys, 2003–2008.

Low birthweight incidence in Africa and Asia and in countries with the highest rates

Percentage of infants weighing less than 2,500 grams at birth

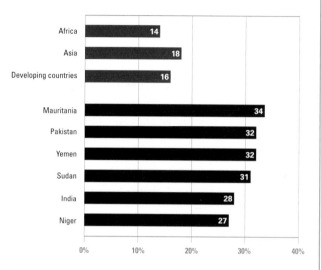

Note: Estimates are based on data collected in 2003 and later with the exception of the Sudan (1999) and Yemen (1997).

Source: MICS, DHS and other national surveys, 2003–2008.

Newborns not weighed in Africa and Asia and in countries with the highest rates

Percentage of infants not weighed at birth

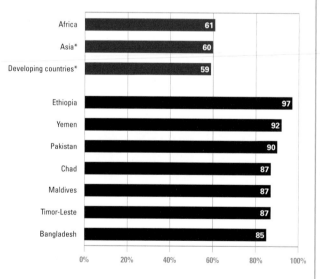

* Excludes China.

Note: Estimates are based on data collected 2003 and later with the exception of Maldives (2001) and Yemen (1997).

Source: MICS, DHS and other national surveys, 2003–2008.

Micronutrient deficiencies

Vitamin and mineral deficiencies are highly prevalent throughout the developing world. The status of vitamin A, iron and iodine deficiencies are highlighted below, but other deficiencies such as zinc and folate are also common.

Vitamin A deficiency remains a significant public health challenge across Africa and Asia and in some countries of South America. An estimated 33 per cent (190 million) of preschool-age children and 15 per cent (19 million) of pregnant women do not have enough vitamin A in their daily diet, and can be classified as vitamin A deficient. The highest prevalence and numbers are found in Africa and some parts of Asia, where more than 40 per cent of preschool-age children are estimated to be vitamin A deficient.[22]

Iron deficiency affects about 25 per cent of the world's population, most of them children of preschool-age and women. It causes anaemia, and the highest proportions of preschool-age children suffering from anaemia are in Africa (68 per cent).[23]

Iodine deficiency, unlike many other nutrition problems, affects both developed and developing countries. Although most people are now protected through the consumption of iodized salt, the proportion of the population affected by iodine deficiency is highest in Europe (52 per cent). Africa is also affected, with 42 per cent of the population assessed as deficient.[24]

4. COVERAGE OF INTERVENTIONS TO IMPROVE NUTRITION

Infant and young child feeding

Optimal infant and young child feeding entails the initiation of breastfeeding within one hour of birth; exclusive breastfeeding for the first six months of the child's life; and continued breastfeeding for two years or more, together with safe, age-appropriate feeding of solid, semi-solid and soft foods starting at 6 months of age.

While infant feeding practices need to be strengthened overall, increasing the rates of early initiation of breastfeeding and of exclusive breastfeeding is critical to improving child survival and development. Less than 40 per cent of all infants in the developing world receive the benefits of immediate initiation of breastfeeding. Similarly, just 37 per cent of children under 6 months of age are exclusively breastfed. Less than 60 per cent of children 6–9 months old receive solid, semi-solid or soft foods while being breastfed. In addition, the quality of the food received is often inadequate, providing insufficient protein, fat or micronutrients for optimal growth and development.

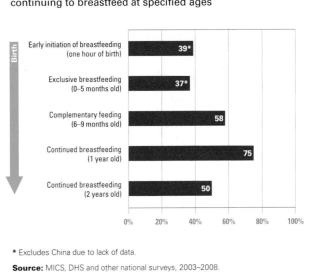

Continuum of infant feeding practices

Percentage of children in the developing world put to the breast within one hour of delivery; exclusively breastfed; both breastfed and receiving complementary foods; and continuing to breastfeed at specified ages

* Excludes China due to lack of data.

Source: MICS, DHS and other national surveys, 2003–2008.

Data indicate that as children develop and complementary foods are introduced, levels of continued breastfeeding are high (75 per cent) at around 1 year of age but decrease to 50 per cent by age 2.

Progress in exclusive breastfeeding rates

Trends in the percentage of infants under 6 months old who are exclusively breastfed

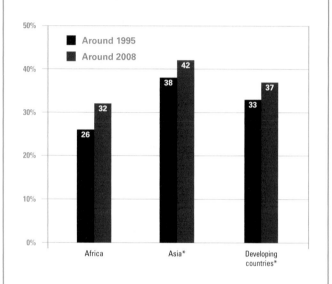

■ Around 1995
■ Around 2008

Africa: 26, 32
Asia*: 38, 42
Developing countries*: 33, 37

* Excludes China due to lack of data.

Note: Analysis is based on a subset of 88 countries with trend data, including 83 developing countries, covering 73 per cent of births in the developing world.

Source: MICS, DHS and other national surveys, around 1995 to around 2008.

Exclusive breastfeeding

In the developing world, less than 40 per cent of infants under 6 months old receive the benefits of exclusive breastfeeding. The rate is particularly low in Africa, where less than one third of infants under 6 months old are exclusively breastfed.

Over the past 10–15 years exclusive breastfeeding rates have increased in many countries of Africa and Asia. In the developing world as a whole, however, progress has been modest, from 33 per cent around 1995 to 37 per cent around 2008.

Evidence from a variety of countries indicates that marked improvements in exclusive breastfeeding are possible if supported by effective regulatory frameworks and guidelines, and when comprehensive programmatic approaches are at scale.

Exclusive breastfeeding rates are very low and stunting prevalence is high in several countries that have experienced emergencies and longer-term challenges, such as Chad, Côte d'Ivoire, Djibouti and the Niger. In these countries, urgent actions are needed to promote and support exclusive breastfeeding in order to reduce the rate of infectious diseases and ensure optimal infant nutrition.

Exclusive breastfeeding rates

Percentage of infants under 6 months old who are exclusively breastfed

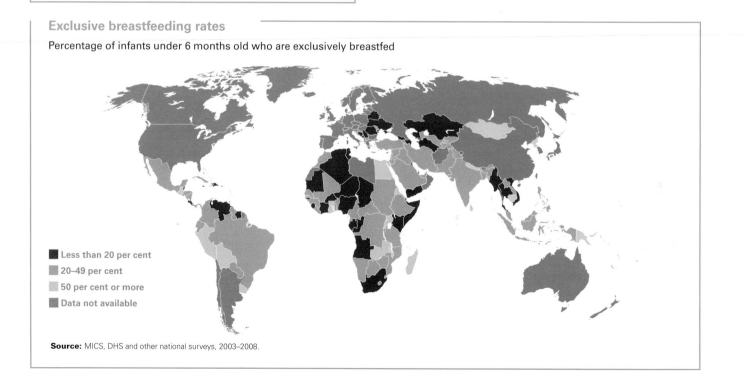

■ Less than 20 per cent
■ 20–49 per cent
■ 50 per cent or more
■ Data not available

Source: MICS, DHS and other national surveys, 2003–2008.

Exclusive breastfeeding rates in Africa and Asia and in countries with both high stunting prevalence and very low exclusive breastfeeding rates

Percentage of infants under 6 months old who are exclusively breastfed

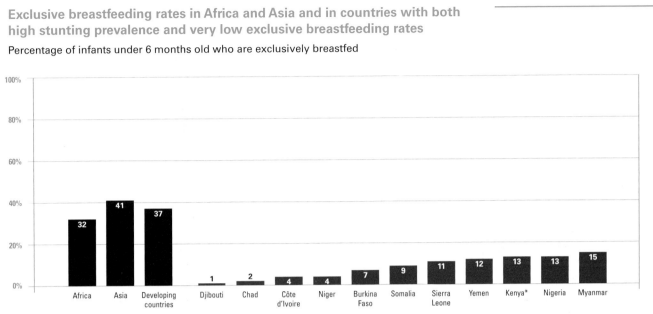

* See box below for recent developments in Kenya.

Note: Countries in this chart have a stunting prevalence of 30% or higher and an exclusive breastfeeding rate of 15% or lower. Stunting prevalence is estimated according to the WHO Child Growth Standards, except for Burkina Faso, Chad and Kenya, where it is estimated according to the NCHS/WHO reference population.

Source: MICS, DHS and other national surveys, 2003–2008.

Integrated approaches to improving infant and young child feeding in Kenya

The exclusive breastfeeding rate for children under 6 months old in Kenya remained static at around 13 per cent from 1993 to 2003. But after the Government, supported by UNICEF, established a comprehensive infant and young child feeding (IYCF) programme in 2007, a substantial increase in the rate of exclusive breastfeeding for this age group took place, according to preliminary data from 2008.

The programme in Kenya is based on the comprehensive, multi-level approach to improving exclusive breastfeeding rates that had proved successful in a number of countries in sub-Saharan Africa and elsewhere. An assessment of people's knowledge, attitudes and practices towards infant and young child feeding guided programme development and laid the foundation for communication and advocacy addressing the challenges to infant feeding in the context of HIV.

Government, non-governmental organizations, and bilateral and multilateral stakeholders then developed a comprehensive IYCF strategy addressing action at the national level, including policy and legislation, at the health-services level and at the community level. Guidelines and training materials were created for use in national capacity and service development, including in maternity facilities, during various maternal and child health contacts, and within communities.

In 2008, the first full year of the programme's implementation, 25 per cent of all health and nutrition service providers and community health workers in most provinces were trained in integrated IYCF counselling. Infant feeding practices in 60 per cent of the country's public hospitals were assessed based on Baby-Friendly Hospital Initiative standards. Communication messages on the benefits of exclusive breastfeeding were broadcast nationwide. The package of services delivered as part of the response to emergency situations emphasized IYCF.

Improved support for infant and young child feeding reached 73 per cent of women attending antenatal care or services to prevent mother-to-child transmission (PMTCT) of HIV in 2008, or an estimated 1.1 million out of the 1.5 million pregnant and lactating women in Kenya. The approach has not only strengthened the crucial infant feeding aspect of PMTCT, it also extended IYCF counselling and communication to the general population.

Non-governmental organizations and the United States President's Emergency Plan for AIDS Relief (PEPFAR) partners implemented the initial phase of IYCF activities; the package of ICYF activities is now being expanded as part of the PEPFAR programme. Within the next two to three years, high coverage of the various activities is anticipated in all provinces.

Sources: UNICEF Kenya Country Office, 'Annual Report 2008' (internal document) and Demographic and Health Surveys, 1993, 1998 and 2003.

Early initiation of breastfeeding

Only 39 per cent of newborns in the developing world are put to the breast within one hour of birth. The rate is especially low in Asia, at 31 per cent.

There is growing evidence of the benefits to mother and child of early initiation of breastfeeding, preferably within the first hour after birth. Early initiation of breastfeeding contributes to reducing overall neonatal mortality.[25] It ensures that skin-to-skin contact is made early on, an important factor in preventing hypothermia and establishing the bond between mother and child. Early initiation of breastfeeding also reduces a mother's risk of post-partum haemorrhage, one of the leading causes of maternal mortality. Colostrum, the milk produced by the mother during the first post-partum days, provides protective antibodies and essential nutrients, acting as a first immunization for newborns, strengthening their immune system and reducing the chances of death in the neonatal period.[26]

In a subset of countries with available data, the low proportions of early initiation of breastfeeding contrast with substantially higher proportions of infants who are delivered by a skilled health professional and of infants whose mothers received antenatal care at least once from a skilled health professional. This gap constitutes a lost opportunity and highlights the critical need to improve the content and quality of counselling by health-care providers.

Complementary feeding

In the developing world, 58 per cent of infants aged 6–9 months old receive complementary foods while continuing to be breastfed. These data do not reflect the quality of the complementary foods received. Meeting minimum standards of dietary quality is a challenge in many developing-country settings, especially in areas where household food security is poor, and it has often not been given enough emphasis. Children may not receive complementary foods at the right age (often either too early or too late), are not fed frequently enough during the day, or the quality of the food may be inadequate. New programming options are now available to meet this challenge.

Complementary feeding is the most effective intervention that can significantly reduce stunting during the first two years of life.[27] A comprehensive programme approach to improving complementary feeding includes counselling for caregivers on feeding and care practices and on the optimal use of locally available foods, improving access to quality foods for poor families through social protection schemes and safety nets, and the provision of micronutrients and fortified food supplements when needed.

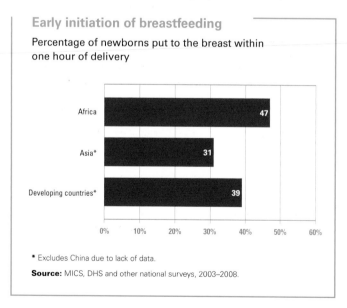

Early initiation of breastfeeding

Percentage of newborns put to the breast within one hour of delivery

* Excludes China due to lack of data.
Source: MICS, DHS and other national surveys, 2003–2008.

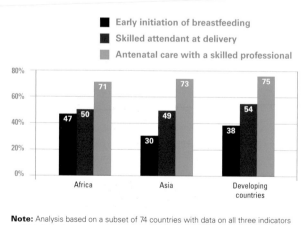

Health-system contacts are not resulting in early initiation of breastfeeding

Percentage of infants who were put to the breast within one hour of birth; percentage of births attended by a skilled health professional; and percentage of pregnant mothers with at least one antenatal care visit with a skilled health professional

Note: Analysis based on a subset of 74 countries with data on all three indicators available from the same survey.
Source: MICS, DHS and other national surveys, 2003–2008.

Recently adopted new indicators for infant and young child feeding (especially the 'minimum acceptable diet' indicator reflecting both frequency of feeding and dietary diversity) emphasize the importance of quality of food and allow for better assessment of complementary feeding practices.

Vitamin A supplementation

Vitamin A is essential for a well-functioning immune system; its deficiency increases the risk of mortality significantly. In 2008, 71 per cent of all children 6–59 months old in developing countries were fully protected against vitamin A deficiency with two doses of vitamin A. Coverage of 85 per cent for the least developed countries highlights the success of programmes in reaching the most vulnerable populations.

In 2008, 22 out of 34 least developed countries with data had surpassed the 80 per cent target of full coverage of vitamin A supplementation. Service provided through integrated child health events has helped to ensure high coverage in a large number of these countries, where weak health systems would otherwise not have reached children. In 2008, integrated child health events were the most effective platform for delivery of vitamin A supplements, resulting in more than 80 per cent coverage on average.[28] Nearly three quarters of the 20 countries with the highest number of deaths among children under 5 years old achieved more than 80 per cent full coverage of vitamin A supplementation.

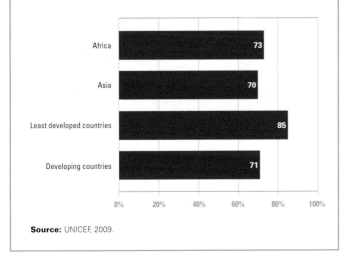

Vitamin A supplementation coverage

Percentage of children 6–59 months old reached with two doses of vitamin A in 2008, in 56 countries with national programmes for which final data were available in July 2009

Source: UNICEF, 2009.

Reaching children with vitamin A in Bihar, India

Vitamin A deficiency is widespread throughout India, but particularly so in rural India, where up to 62 per cent of preschool-age children are deficient, according to the latest estimates. Moreover, the high prevalence of wasting (20 per cent), stunting (48 per cent) and anaemia (70 per cent) in children under 5 years old indicates widespread nutritional deprivation.

India's national policy recommends that all children 9–59 months old be given preventive vitamin A supplementation twice yearly to reduce the risk of blindness, infection, undernutrition and death associated with vitamin A deficiency, particularly among the most vulnerable children. Many states in India have put the fight against vitamin A deficiency on a 'war footing', and Bihar State – one of the poorest in India – is at the forefront of this battle.

The Government of Bihar, in partnership with UNICEF, the Micronutrient Initiative and others, supports a strategy to increase coverage of vitamin A supplementation beyond the levels achieved through routine contact with the health system. The goal is to reach out to all children, beginning with children in socially excluded groups, scheduled castes and minority groups in which undernutrition and mortality rates are significantly higher than among children outside these groups.

District planning has been a crucial tool. More than 11,000 health centres and 80,000 *anganwadis*, or child development centres, that serve as core distribution sites for vitamin A supplementation in Bihar have been mapped out, and more than 3,400 temporary sites have been organized to deliver vitamin A supplements within small, isolated communities. Front-line health and nutrition workers and community volunteers in the 38 districts of Bihar have been trained to administer preventive vitamin A syrup to children and to counsel mothers on how to improve the vitamin A content of their children's diet.

The latest coverage data indicate that in the first semester of 2009, Bihar's vitamin A supplementation programme reached 13.4 million children 9–59 months old, protecting 95 per cent of children in this age group against the devastating consequences of vitamin A deficiency.

The Government of Bihar is demonstrating that it is feasible to undertake inclusive programming for child nutrition and to reach children who are traditionally excluded from services when efforts are made to understand who these children are and where they live – and when political decisions are made to assign the human and programme resources needed to reach them.

Sources: Official statistics provided to UNICEF by the Government of Bihar, October 2009 (internal documents).

Vitamin A supplementation coverage rates show dramatic increases in a relatively short period of time. In Africa, full coverage of vitamin A supplementation has increased fivefold since 2000, due largely to the introduction of biannual child health days, the main platform for vitamin A supplement distribution in many African countries. Importantly, coverage more than doubled in the least developed countries, rising from 41 per cent in 2000 to 88 per cent in 2008, demonstrating that this life-saving intervention is reaching children in countries where it is most needed.

Progress in vitamin A supplementation coverage

Percentage of children 6–59 months old reached with two doses of vitamin A, 2000–2008

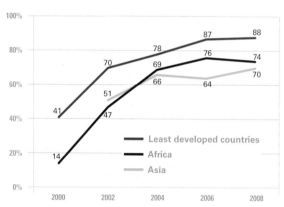

Note: Vitamin A supplementation two-dose (full coverage) trends are based on a subset of 16 African countries and 18 least developed countries with data in even years between 2000 and 2008 and on a subset of 11 Asian countries with data in even years between 2002 and 2008. The trend line for Asia begins in 2002 because of a lack of data for trend analysis prior to that.

Source: UNICEF, 2009.

Universal salt iodization

Iodine deficiency can be easily prevented by ensuring that salt consumed by households is adequately iodized. The most recent data indicate that 36 countries have reached the target of at least 90 per cent of households using adequately iodized salt. This represents an increase from 21 countries in 2002, when the universal salt iodization goal was endorsed at the United Nations General Assembly Special Session on Children. Despite this significant progress, about 41 million newborns a year remain unprotected from the enduring consequences of brain damage associated with iodine deficiency.

Some 72 per cent of all households in developing countries now consume adequately iodized salt. About 73 per cent of households in Asia and 60 per cent in Africa consume adequately iodized salt. Africa's relatively high rate is largely due to high coverage in two populous countries – Nigeria (with 97 per cent coverage) and the Democratic Republic of the Congo (79 per cent) – which masks the low coverage in many less populous countries of the region.

125 countries are now implementing and reporting on salt iodization programmes, an increase of 39 per cent in just seven years

Number of countries implementing and reporting on salt iodization programmes, 2002–2009, by level of coverage

	Number of countries		Change 2002–2009	
	Reported in			
	2002	2009	Number of countries	Percentage
Countries with more than 90% coverage	21	36	+15	+71%
Countries with 70–89% coverage	17	27	+10	+59%
Countries with 50–69% coverage	17	22	+5	+29%
Countries with 20–49% coverage	22	28	+6	+27%
Countries with less than 20% coverage	13	12	-1	-8%
Total number of countries implementing and reporting on programmes	90	125	+35	+39%

Source: The 'reported in 2002' column represents UNICEF data published in *Progress Since the World Summit for Children: A statistical review* (2002). The 'reported in 2009' column represents UNICEF data published in the statistical tables accompanying *The State of the World's Children Special Edition: Celebrating 20 Years of the Convention on the Rights of the Child* (2009).

Iodized salt consumption

Percentage of households consuming adequately iodized salt

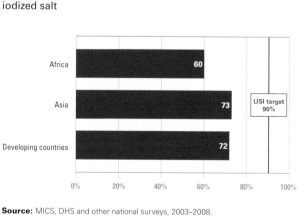

Source: MICS, DHS and other national surveys, 2003–2008.

Increases in excess of 30 percentage points over the past decade have occurred in 19 countries where the current levels of household consumption of adequately iodized salt exceed 70 per cent. These marked improvements are a product of a unique combination of innovative public policies, private-sector initiative and civic commitment. Thirteen of these countries have improved their coverage by more than 50 percentage points, indicating that the goal of universal salt iodization can be attained – even at the global level – if efforts are similarly strengthened among countries that are lagging.

Government commitment helps eliminate iodine deficiency in Nigeria

In the 1980s, iodine deficiency was a significant public health concern in Nigeria, with a total goitre rate of 67 per cent in 1988. This left many children at risk of mental and cognitive impairment. To combat this public health problem, the Government, in collaboration with UNICEF, launched the Universal Salt Iodization programme. This initiative is now managed by the National Agency for Food and Drug Administration and Control in collaboration with the Standards Organization of Nigeria, the National Planning Commission and the Ministry of Health.

At the time the Universal Salt Iodization programme started in 1993, only 40 per cent of households consumed adequately iodized salt. The programme has achieved tremendous success, with 97 per cent of households now consuming adequately iodized salt and with factories producing 90–100 per cent iodized salt. The goitre rate has plummeted, to about 6 per cent in 2007.

By 2007, Nigeria became the first country in Africa to receive recognition by the Network for Sustained Elimination of Iodine Deficiency. Nigeria's success in eliminating iodine deficiency disorder can be attributed to the commitment of the Government and the salt industry, effective legislation and strong enforcement.

Sources: *Universal Salt Iodization in Nigeria: Process, successes and lessons,* Government of Nigeria, Ministry of Health, and UNICEF, Abuja, 2007.

Outstanding improvements in the use of iodized salt

Trends in the percentage of households consuming adequately iodized salt, selected countries and territories

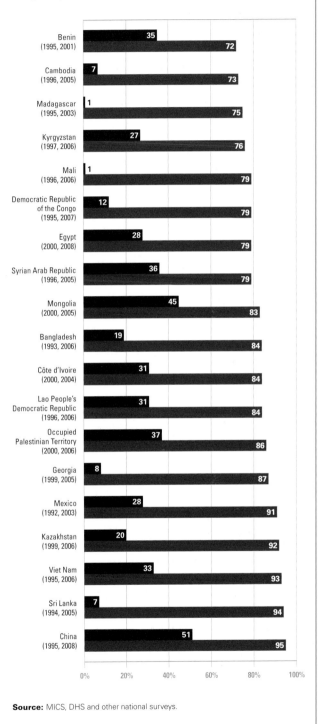

Source: MICS, DHS and other national surveys.

Fortification of staple foods and condiments

Along with the iodization of salt, adding such vitamins and minerals as iron, zinc, vitamin A and folic acid to staple foods, complementary foods and condiments is a cost-effective way to improve the vitamin and mineral intake of the overall population, including women of reproductive age and children. As of March 2009, roughly 30 per cent of the world's wheat flour produced in large roller mills was fortified, while 57 countries had legislation or decrees mandating fortification of one or more types of flour with either iron or folic acid.[29] Although many foods, such as fats, oils and margarine, have been fortified for years in some countries, this approach has not yet been scaled up in many lower-income countries. Through increased efforts by various partnerships and alliances, it is expected that food fortification will continue to gain momentum.

Multiple micronutrient supplementation/home fortification

Among products recently developed to provide iron and other vitamins and minerals to young children and women of reproductive age, multiple micronutrient powders (MNPs) are considered particularly promising; studies have found they may reduce anaemia in young children by as much as 45 per cent.[30] MNP sachets contain a blend of vitamins and minerals in powdered form that can be sprinkled onto home-prepared foods, enabling families without access to commercially fortified foods to add micronutrients directly to their diets. There is emerging evidence that MNPs can contribute to improving complementary feeding practices if programmes are designed with that goal in mind.[31]

Multi-micronutrients for Mongolian children

In recent years, multiple micronutrient powders that can improve vitamin and mineral intake among infants over 6 months old and young children have become available globally to address what appeared to be an intractable, widespread public health problem of iron-deficiency anaemia. The powders can contain 5–15 vitamins and minerals (such as iron, and vitamins A and D), are relatively tasteless, and are safe, easy to use and acceptable to caregivers. They cost about US$0.03 per sachet (one child typically gets 60–90 sachets per year), and there is sufficient commercial supply to meet programme needs.

Mongolia is among the many countries that are introducing and scaling up the use of MNPs as part of an integrated approach to improve young child feeding and reduce stunting and anaemia. The Mongolian effort, part of a comprehensive national nutrition strategy to tackle chronic undernutrition, is also a way to address the nutritional fallout from the economic instability and chronic food shortages that have plagued the country in the past few years.

The country's approach builds on an experience of distributing MNPs to children 6–36 months old to reduce anaemia and vitamin D deficiency. At the onset of that distribution, in 2001, the baseline prevalence of anaemia was around 42 per cent. Children received MNPs via a community distribution model and also had biweekly visits by community workers supported by the Ministry of Health.

One year into the programme, 13,000 children, or more than 80 per cent of those targeted, had received multi-micronutrient powders, and anaemia was reduced to half of baseline levels. With technical and financial support from the Asian Development Bank, Mongolia plans to expand the programme to reach some 15,000 children 6–24 months old (or 22 per cent of all children in this age range) by targeting provinces based on poverty levels, geographical access and health indicators.

Sources: 'Micronutrient Sprinkles for Use in Infants and Young Children: Guidelines on recommendations for use and program monitoring and evaluation', Sprinkles Global Health Initiative, Toronto, December 2008; and Schauer, C., et al., 'Process Evaluation of the Distribution of Micronutrient Sprinkles in over 10,000 Mongolian Infants Using a Non-Governmental Organization (NGO) Program Model', abstract presented at the International Nutritional Anemia Consultative Group Symposium, Marrakech, February 2003, p.42.

5. EFFECTIVE INTERVENTIONS TO IMPROVE NUTRITION

The period in the life cycle from the mother's pregnancy to the child's second birthday provides a critical window of opportunity in which interventions to improve maternal and child undernutrition can have a positive impact on young children's prospects for survival, growth and development, especially in countries with a high burden of undernutrition.

A package of effective nutrition interventions has widely been agreed upon by experts and programme partners. It includes interventions in three key areas:

- Maternal nutrition during pregnancy and lactation.
- Initiation of breastfeeding within the first hour after birth, exclusive breastfeeding for the first 6 months, and continued breastfeeding up to at least 24 months of age.
- Adequate complementary feeding from 6 months onward, and micronutrient interventions as needed.

Successful programming in these areas will lead to marked reductions in the levels of chronic undernutrition in young children.

Effective interventions for the treatment of severe acute malnutrition in both emergency and non-emergency settings include the use of ready-to-use therapeutic foods and adequate treatment of complications, and, for management of moderate acute malnutrition, the use of various supplementary foods. These interventions need to be implemented at scale together with strategies to improve care and feeding practices.

Given the close link between undernutrition and infections, the implementation at scale of key interventions to prevent and treat infections will contribute to better nutrition as well as reduced mortality. Such interventions include immunization, improved hygiene and hand washing, sanitation (including the elimination of open defecation) and access to clean drinking water, use of improved oral rehydration salts and therapeutic zinc to treat diarrhoea, the prevention and treatment of malaria, and the treatment of pneumonia with antibiotics.

Reducing acute malnutrition in the Niger

Unacceptable levels of malnutrition due to drought, recurring food crises, poor feeding practices and inadequate access to health services have plagued the Niger for years. In 2005, nutrition surveys documented the prevalence of global acute malnutrition (severe and moderate acute malnutrition combined) above emergency thresholds of 15 per cent in several regions, triggering a major emergency response by the Government and the international community. One result was a significant drop in prevalence to 10 per cent in 2006.

A vital component of the successful effort was a shift to programming approaches that allowed for many more affected individuals to be treated. A decentralized, community-based approach to treating acute malnutrition was used for the first time. Children with severe acute malnutrition were treated in their homes using ready-to-use therapeutic food. Moderate acute malnutrition was treated with a range of products, including the traditional fortified blended flour as well as an oil-based ready-to-use supplementary food. Some partners also expanded nutrition treatment programmes to include prevention of acute malnutrition through the large-scale distribution of supplementary food products.

The number of facilities in the Niger where treatment for severe acute malnutrition was provided jumped from 75 in 2005 to 941 in 2007. The increased demand for therapeutic and supplementary food products prompted creation of a local production facility that is increasingly meeting the demand.

Although significant progress has been made since 2005 in the Niger's ability to effectively treat severely acutely malnourished children through the community-based approach, the prevalence of acute malnutrition remains high. The challenge is to scale up such preventive practices as breastfeeding and improving complementary feeding, which would significantly improve child nutrition and contribute to lowering the numbers of children with moderate or severe acute malnutrition.

Sources: *Community-based Management of Severe Acute Malnutrition: A joint statement by the World Health Organization, the World Food Programme, the United Nations System Standing Committee on Nutrition and the United Nations Children's Fund,* WHO, WFP, SCN and UNICEF, Geneva, Rome and New York, May 2007; and 'Humanitarian Action Niger', UNICEF, New York, June 2006.

Community-based management of severe acute malnutrition in Malawi

In Malawi each year, there are an estimated 59,000 children with severe acute malnutrition. Around 59 per cent of these children are currently being treated, at a recovery rate of more than 75 per cent, which makes Malawi a leader globally in achieving results in the management of severe acute malnutrition. A vital component of Malawi's success has been the introduction of community-based management of the condition.

Poor nutritional status has been a chronic problem in Malawi. In addition to endemic diseases and the AIDS epidemic, from 2001–2006 Malawi experienced persistent episodes of food shortage and other humanitarian crises. The rate of global acute malnutrition nationally was 6.2 per cent in 2005; four districts had rates above 10 per cent. Prior to 2006, management of severe acute malnutrition took place on an inpatient basis in paediatric wards and in nutrition rehabilitation units using the milk-based therapeutic preparations.

In 2002, however, the non-governmental organizations Concern Worldwide and Valid International introduced an innovative approach using ready-to-use therapeutic food to increase coverage of treatment for severe acute malnutrition. The initiative, anchored at the district level, encourages communities to identify severely undernourished children before they require inpatient care. Effective treatment is then given on a weekly basis at local health structures or at distribution sites within a day's walk of people's homes. Inpatient care is available for complicated cases.

These efforts led to expanded coverage of effective treatment, reaching 74 per cent of those in need, compared to 25 per cent for the traditional approach. After extending the initiative to additional districts following a 2004 review, the model was adopted as a national strategy in 2006, and its gradual scale-up and integration into the primary-health-care system began. By March 2009, the programme had been scaled up to 330 outpatient and 96 inpatient sites in all of the country's 27 districts, and it is expected to eventually reach all health facilities in the country.

Sources: *Community-based Management of Severe Acute Malnutrition: A joint statement by the World Health Organization, the World Food Programme, the United Nations System Standing Committee on Nutrition, and the United Nations Children's Fund*, WHO, WFP, SCN and UNICEF, Geneva, Rome and New York, May 2007; and UNICEF Malawi Country Office Annual Reports and other internal documents.

In many countries and communities, households face periods of seasonal food shortage, or adequate nutritious food may be unavailable to families on a continual basis. This situation needs to be addressed in order to ensure adequate maternal nutrition and complementary feeding for infants and young children, as well as to sustain reductions in undernutrition over the long term. Interventions include measures to improve agricultural production and to increase food availability through social protection schemes and food distribution programmes.

The table on the following pages offers detailed information on the priority interventions for the prevention of undernutrition and the treatment of severe and moderate acute malnutrition to be delivered at stages of the life cycle between the woman's pregnancy and the child's second birthday. Some of these preventive actions should begin in adolescence, before the woman becomes pregnant, and continue after the child reaches 24 months of age. Many of these interventions endeavour to change behaviour and will depend on the successful implementation of large-scale communication strategies.

Adequate nutrition is also of key importance for children more than 2 years old, and interventions such as vitamin A supplementation, zinc treatment for diarrhoea, management of acute malnutrition, and communication and counselling on the prevention of both undernutrition and overweight are also crucial for these children.

Priority interventions for the prevention of undernutrition and the treatment of severe and moderate acute malnutrition

Life cycle stage	
Adolescence/pre-pregnancy	
Interventions for the mother	**Justification/evidence**
Iron and folic acid supplements or multiple micronutrient supplementation, and deworming	Reduces iron deficiency and other micronutrient deficiencies, and anaemia in pregnancy
Food fortification with folic acid, iron, vitamin A, zinc and iodine	Reduces micronutrient deficiencies; prevents neural tube defects and negative effects associated with iodine deficiency in early pregnancy
Pregnancy	
Interventions for the mother	**Justification/evidence**
Iron and folic acid supplements and deworming	Reduces micronutrient deficiency, pregnancy complications, maternal mortality and low birthweight
Multi-micronutrient supplementation	Reduces micronutrient deficiency; contributes to improving birthweight and child growth and development
Iodized salt consumed as table salt and/or as food-grade salt (used in food processing)	Improves fetal development, cognition and intelligence in infant; reduces risks of complications during pregnancy and delivery; prevents goitre, miscarriages, stillbirth and cretinism
Treatment of night blindness in pregnancy	Controls maternal vitamin A deficiency and subsequent deficiency in early infancy
Fortified food (with iron, folate, zinc, vitamin A, iodine)	Reduces micronutrient deficiency and birth defects
Improved use of locally available foods to ensure increased intake of important nutrients	Reduces wasting and micronutrient deficiencies; contributes to reducing low birthweight
Fortified food supplements (e.g., corn-soya blends, lipid-based nutrient supplements) for undernourished women	Reduces wasting and micronutrient deficiencies; contributes to reducing low birthweight
Birth	
Interventions for the infant	**Justification/evidence**
Initiation of breastfeeding within 1 hour (including colostrum feeding)	Contributes to reduction of neonatal deaths
Less than 6 months	
Interventions for the mother	**Justification/evidence**
Vitamin A supplement in first 8 weeks after delivery	Repletion of maternal vitamin A status improves vitamin A content of breastmilk; contributes to reducing vitamin A deficiency in infants and reduces infections
Multi-micronutrient supplementation	Reduces iron and other micronutrient deficiencies in mother; improves quality of breastmilk
Improved use of locally available foods, fortified foods, micronutrient supplementation/home fortification and food supplements for undernourished women	Prevents maternal undernutrition; helps maintain ability to breastfeed and ensure high-quality breastmilk
Interventions for the infant	**Justification/evidence**
Exclusive breastfeeding	Assures optimal nutrient intake and prevents childhood disease and death
Appropriate feeding of HIV-exposed infants	Contributes to reducing mother-to-child transmission of HIV and to reducing infant mortality

Priority interventions for the prevention of undernutrition and the treatment of severe and moderate acute malnutrition (continued)

Life cycle stage	
6–23 months	
Interventions for the mother	**Justification/evidence**
Improved use of locally available foods, fortified foods and food supplements for undernourished women	Helps maintain breastfeeding and ensure high-quality breastmilk, as well as prevent maternal undernutrition
Hand washing with soap	Helps reduce diarrhoea and associated undernutrition in the child
Interventions for the young child	**Justification/evidence**
Timely, adequate, safe and appropriate complementary feeding (including improved use of local foods, multi-micronutrient supplementation, lipid-based nutrient supplements and fortified complementary foods)	Prevents and decreases underweight, stunting, wasting and micronutrient deficiency and contributes to survival and development; also contributes to reducing childhood obesity
Continued breastfeeding	Provides significant source of nutrients; protects from infections
Appropriate feeding of HIV-exposed infants	Contributes to reducing mother-to-child transmission of HIV and reducing child mortality
Zinc treatment for diarrhoea	Reduces duration and severity of diarrhoea and subsequent episodes; reduces mortality
Iodized salt consumed as table salt and/or as food-grade salt (used in food processing)	Improves brain development; prevents motor and hearing deficits
Vitamin A supplementation and deworming	Contributes to reducing anaemia, vitamin A deficiency and undernutrition, and to reducing child mortality
Management of severe acute malnutrition	Contributes to reducing child mortality
Management of moderate acute malnutrition	Prevents progression to severe acute malnutrition and contributes to reducing child mortality
Hand washing with soap	Helps reduce diarrhoea and associated undernutrition
24–59 months	
Interventions for the young child	**Justification/evidence**
Vitamin A supplementation with deworming	Contributes to reducing anaemia, vitamin A deficiency and undernutrition and to reducing child mortality
Multi-micronutrient powder or fortified foods for young children	Reduces iron and zinc deficiency
Iodized salt consumed as table salt and/or as food-grade salt (used in food processing)	Improves brain development; prevents motor and hearing deficits
Management of severe acute malnutrition	Contributes to reducing child mortality
Management of moderate acute malnutrition	Prevents progression to severe acute malnutrition and contributes to reducing child mortality
Hand washing with soap	Helps reduce diarrhoea and associated undernutrition

Sources: Policy and guideline recommendations based on WHO and other UN agencies; publications in *The Lancet*; Edmond, Karen M., et al., 'Delayed Breastfeeding Initiation Increases Risk of Neonatal Mortality', *Pediatrics*, vol. 117, no. 3, March 2006, pp. 3380–3386; Singh, Kiran, and Purnima Srivasta, 'The Effect of Colostrum on Infant Mortality: Urban-rural differentials', *Health and Population*, vol. 15, no. 3–4, July–December 1992, pp. 94–100; Mullany, Luke C., et al., 'Breastfeeding Patterns, Time to Initiation and Mortality Risk Among Newborns in Southern Nepal', *The Journal of Nutrition*, vol. 138, March 2008, pp. 599–603; Ramakrishnan, Usha, et al., 'Effects of Micronutrients on Growth of Children Under 5 Years of Age: Meta-analyses of single and multiple nutrient interventions', *The American Journal of Clinical Nutrition*, vol. 89, no. 1, January 2009, pp. 191–203.

6. UNDERLYING CAUSES OF UNDERNUTRITION: POVERTY, DISPARITIES AND OTHER SOCIAL FACTORS

Poverty, inequity, low maternal education and women's social status are among the underlying factors that need to be taken into consideration and addressed in order to reduce undernutrition in a sustained manner.

Poverty

The relationship between poverty and nutrition is two-sided: Economic growth, when it contributes to lowering the prevalence of poverty and food insecurity, can also lead to reduced undernutrition, albeit at a slow pace.[32] Nutrition is one of the key elements for human capital formation, which in turn represents one of the fundamental drivers of economic growth.[33]

But economic growth does not necessarily translate to better and equitable outcomes for all individuals in society, and the nutritional status of a population does not always depend on national development, prosperity or economic growth.

Maternal and child nutrition is the result of a wide variety of factors, reflecting the quality of public health systems, caring practices in households and communities, society's ability to deal with poverty, food insecurity for disadvantaged groups, the capacities of social justice and welfare systems, and the effectiveness of broader economic and social policies. Nutrition status can therefore be improved even when economic growth remains limited.[34] In fact, addressing undernutrition helps to halt the intergenerational transmission of poverty.

Equity

Equity issues are important when assessing progress on nutrition globally. Analysing disparities in equity can lead to a better understanding of the causes of undernutrition, and it can help identify and target interventions for the most vulnerable populations within a country or region as part of a multi-sectoral nutrition strategy.

Although a number of countries have made progress combating child undernutrition, closer scrutiny using an 'equity lens' reveals large inequities. The Plurinational State of Bolivia, for example, halved stunting prevalence among children under 5 years old between 1989 and 2003, but children in the poorest households are nearly six times as likely to be stunted as children in the richest households. In Peru, children in the poorest households are 11 times more likely to be stunted than children in the richest households.[35]

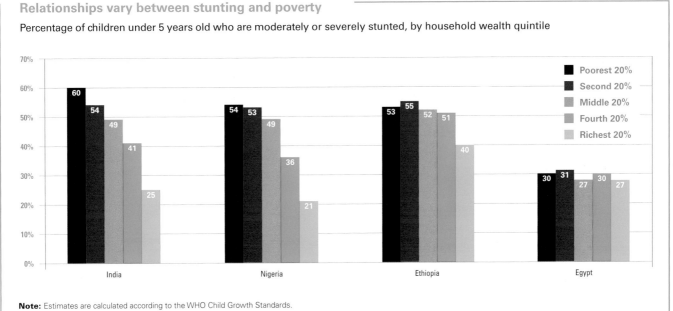

Relationships vary between stunting and poverty

Percentage of children under 5 years old who are moderately or severely stunted, by household wealth quintile

Note: Estimates are calculated according to the WHO Child Growth Standards.

Source: India: National Family Health Survey (2005–2006), Nigeria: DHS (2003), Ethiopia: DHS (2005), Egypt: DHS (2008).

The relationship between stunting and wealth varies significantly across countries. In India and Nigeria, children in the richest households are at a distinct advantage compared to children in other households. This contrasts with Ethiopia, where stunting is widespread – even among children living in the wealthiest households, the prevalence of stunting is high, at 40 per cent – and in Egypt, where stunting prevalence is remarkably similar in all wealth quintiles.

Children in rural areas in the developing world are almost twice as likely to be underweight as children in urban areas.

Gender and social norms

An analysis of nutrition indicators at the global level reveals negligible differences between boys and girls under 5 years old. Similarly, programme coverage and practice data that are disaggregated by sex reveal no significant differences on the basis of gender. But further disaggregation of data from some countries indicates there might be differences in the feeding and care of girls compared to boys, presumably stemming from power relations and social norms that perpetuate discriminatory attitudes and practices. Data in some countries point to the possible effects, such as Bangladeshi boys being significantly taller relative to their age than girls.[36] In sub-Saharan Africa, on the other hand, boys are more likely to be stunted than girls.[37]

Maternal education

Significant disparity in nutritional status also exists in terms of mothers' education and literacy. A number of studies and analyses have found a significant association between low maternal literacy and poor nutrition status of young children. An analysis of survey data from 17 developing countries, for example, confirms a positive association between maternal education and nutritional status in children 3–23 months old, although a large part of these associations is the result of education's strong link to household economics.[38] A study in Pakistan revealed that the majority of infants with signs of undernutrition had mothers with virtually no schooling. The study also observed that the introduction of complementary foods for infants at an appropriate age (6 months) improved when mothers were educated.[39]

Women's social status

In many developing countries, the low status of women is considered to be one of the primary determinants of undernutrition across the life cycle. Women's low status can result in their own health outcomes being compromised, which in turn can lead to lower infant birthweight and may affect the quality of infant care and nutrition. A study in India showed that women with higher autonomy (indicated by access to money and freedom to choose to go to the market) were significantly less likely to have a stunted child when compared with their peers who had less autonomy.[40]

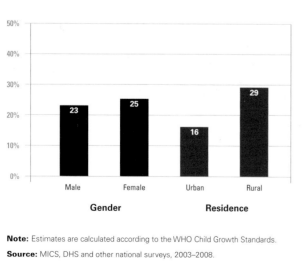

Underweight prevalence, by gender and area of residence

Percentage of children under 5 years old in developing countries who are moderately or severely underweight, by gender and area of residence

	Gender		Residence	
	Male	Female	Urban	Rural
	23	25	16	29

Note: Estimates are calculated according to the WHO Child Growth Standards.

Source: MICS, DHS and other national surveys, 2003–2008.

7. FACTORS FOR GOOD NUTRITION PROGRAMMING

The packages of interventions for the prevention and treatment of undernutrition described in Section 5 of this Overview must be implemented at a large scale if they are to translate to real gains in reducing child undernutrition. Effective programming – based on adequate policies and regulatory frameworks, strong management and functioning service delivery systems, and backed by sufficient resources – is also imperative to achieve a high coverage of service delivery and to effect widespread change in community and household behaviours and practices.

Experience shows that it is entirely feasible to scale up nutrition programmes and achieve marked improvements in caring behaviour and practices, especially when there is strong government leadership and broad supporting partnerships. Over the past 5–10 years, for example, 16 countries have recorded gains of 20 percentage points or more in exclusive breastfeeding rates. Many of these countries face serious development challenges, as well as emergency situations. The implementation of large-scale programmes in these countries was based on national policies and often guided by the WHO-UNICEF Global Strategy for Infant and Young Child Feeding. Country programmes included the adoption and implementation of national legislation on the International Code of Marketing of Breastmilk Substitutes and subsequent World Health Assembly resolutions, as well as maternity protection for working women. Further actions included ensuring that breastfeeding was initiated in maternity facilities (and that no infant formula was given in the facilities), building health worker capacity to offer counselling on infant and young child feeding, and mother-to-mother support groups in the community. These actions were accompanied by communication strategies to promote breastfeeding using multiple channels and messages tailored to the local context.[41]

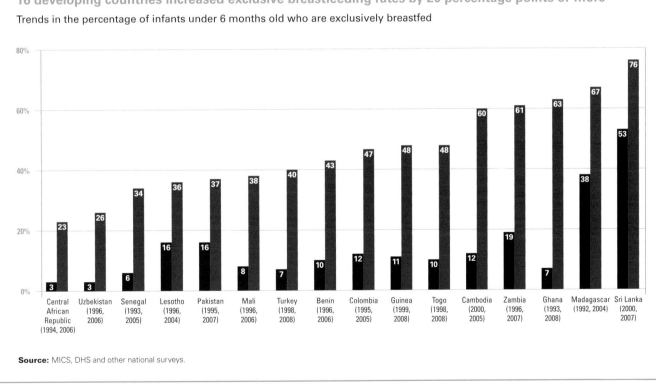

16 developing countries increased exclusive breastfeeding rates by 20 percentage points or more

Trends in the percentage of infants under 6 months old who are exclusively breastfed

Source: MICS, DHS and other national surveys.

The recent global initiative on community-based treatment of severe acute malnutrition is an excellent example of partnership among many organizations working together to reach children with life-saving services not available to them before. A total of 42 countries in Africa, Asia and the Middle East, including countries facing chronic or acute emergencies, have finalized or drafted integrated guidelines and action plans for scale-up and integration within the regular health system.[42] Guidance on planning and implementation has been provided by international partners, and health-worker capacity has been strengthened. In parallel, the production and distribution of therapeutic products has drastically increased, particularly for ready-to-use therapeutic food.[43]

While prioritizing the acceleration of programmes to provide treatment for children with severe acute malnutrition, it is also important to implement actions to prevent it – including measures to expand infant and young child feeding, improve health care and hygiene conditions, and promote food security.

In many countries, integrated child health events have proved effective in delivering vitamin A. This approach – which employs good planning, capacity strengthening and the pooling of resources – allows for wide coverage of a package of interventions in situations where delivery through routine health services is limited.

Integrated child health events improve vitamin A supplementation coverage in Mozambique and Zambia

Many countries are using integrated child health events to significantly increase coverage of selected health and nutrition interventions and to improve equity of coverage. In 2008, Mozambique introduced integrated Child Health Weeks in order to achieve high coverage of this type of essential child survival intervention, particularly in hard-to-reach populations. The Child Health Weeks offer vitamin A supplements, deworming, measles vaccination, nutrition screening, nutrition messages on breastfeeding and distribution of iodized oil supplements. A key feature of these events is that services are offered closer to people's homes.

For the first round of Child Health Weeks in March–April 2008, Mozambique achieved more than 80 per cent coverage of vitamin A supplementation, made possible by integrated, district-level micro-planning, supportive supervision of community-level workers, and monitoring. Integration of the planning of Child Health Weeks into comprehensive district-level planning processes is expected to enhance sustainability. After the first child-health event, post-event coverage analysis identified low-performing districts so that implementation could be improved for subsequent distribution rounds.

Zambia has supported integrated child health events for a decade now, and has achieved progressively high coverage of essential child health and nutrition interventions. Child Health Weeks were initially introduced to increase coverage of interventions such as vitamin A supplementation. Increased demand for services eventually led to expansion of Child Health Weeks to include additional high-impact interventions such as routine childhood vaccinations, health education, promotion of hand washing, nutritional screening, HIV testing, family planning and management of common childhood illnesses.

Given its success in increasing coverage of these interventions, particularly in hard-to-reach areas of the country, the Government has institutionalized Child Health Weeks. In 2008, all but two provinces reported vitamin A and deworming coverage of more than 80 per cent. One recent innovation has the country's leading mobile phone service sending out free text messages urging parents and caregivers to participate.

Sources: UNICEF Mozambique Country Office, 'Annual Report 2008', and UNICEF Zambia Country Office, 'Annual Report 2008' (internal documents).

PROGRAMME SUCCESS FACTORS

1. **Situation analysis:** The starting point in the design of programmes should always be the analysis of the local nutrition situation and its determinants, including household food security, poverty and social issues. This analysis should form the basis for appropriate national policies, adequate legislative frameworks and strategies that ensure the best use of local resources. Policy guidance and technical documentation on international norms already established can facilitate policy design and choice of implementation strategy.

2. **Political commitment and partnership:** Strong and clear government ownership, leadership and commitment are keys to the success of any nutrition programme. Nutrition often falls within the mandate of several departments, so programmes require clear roles and responsibilities; similar clarity and well-coordinated support is required from the international community. The Renewed Efforts Against Childhood Hunger and Undernutrition (REACH) initiative provides a good example of inter-agency collaboration and partnerships to improve nutrition *(see box on the next page)*.

3. **Linkages with other sectors:** The packages of nutrition interventions described in this report need to be implemented in conjunction with relevant health and water/sanitation interventions – particularly those addressing treatment and prevention of the major childhood illnesses closely associated with undernutrition (diarrhoea, pneumonia, malaria, measles, and HIV and AIDS). Better household food security, through strengthened agricultural and social protection programmes, is essential to sustain efforts to improve nutrition.

4. **Capacity-building:** Early initiation of breastfeeding and exclusive breastfeeding can be effectively promoted using various channels at all levels of the primary-health-care system, including antenatal care clinics and traditional birth attendants; home visits by community health workers; immunization and weighing sessions, and sick child consultations; and services to prevent mother-to-child transmission of HIV and provide paediatric AIDS treatment. For health workers to do this work effectively, the reach and coverage of the health system needs to be reviewed, opportunities identified, and knowledge and skills updated and strengthened. Capacity building is therefore critical to the success of nutrition programmes.

5. **Communication and community:** Experience shows that effective large-scale communication campaigns and community involvement are key conditions for programmes that seek to improve child care and nutrition and promote behavioural change. Regular support and counselling of caregivers at the community level in a comprehensive manner, with messaging on feeding, care, hygiene, and disease prevention and treatment, can lead to positive outcomes. For this purpose, many countries successfully rely on community-based volunteers who work closely with official service providers. Strong emphasis on quality implementation of planned activities at the community level includes supportive supervision and continuous monitoring and evaluation with feedback mechanisms. The notion of communities as passive recipients of services is no longer valid; they are active agents for identifying and addressing gaps, assuming responsibilities and ensuring that adequate nutrition is provided for all.

6. **Corporate social responsibility:** The involvement of the private sector can ensure the availability of appropriate and affordable products, such as high-quality foods for complementary feeding and supplementary feeding, and micronutrient-fortified staple foods and supplements. This is an important strategy that can both improve access to quality foods and lead to increased local production. With its extensive access to populations, the private sector also has a role in encouraging behaviour change that promotes healthy lifestyles and good nutrition. In this way, corporate social responsibility can help improve child and maternal nutrition. It is critical that companies comply with the International Code of Marketing of Breastmilk Substitutes and all relevant standards.

7. **Resources:** Nutrition programmes are usually severely under-resourced – despite evidence of their effectiveness. The Copenhagen Consensus 2008, for example, listed nutrition interventions among the most cost-effective actions to tackle some of the world's most pressing challenges. According to the Copenhagen Consensus, a global investment of US$60 million per year for vitamin A and zinc supplementation would yield a return in benefits of US$1 billion.[44] The programme 'A Good Start in Life' in Peru documented a significant reduction in stunting at an annual cost of about US$117 per child.[45] The REACH initiative is estimated to need about US$36 per child per year to implement an integrated programme with cost-effective interventions.[46] Although the cost of programmes will vary widely between countries, depending on many local conditions, these figures provide an indication of the resources required.

Ending child hunger and undernutrition in Mauritania: The REACH partnership

As part of the global REACH effort to end child hunger, Mauritania, along with the Lao People's Democratic Republic, was the site of a pilot project launched in June 2008. REACH – Renewed Efforts Against Child Hunger and Undernutrition – is driven by a partnership between governments, non-governmental and civil society organizations, and the United Nations, with the goal of improving efficiency and coordination of the work to advance children's nutritional status. It aims to accelerate progress towards MDG 1, target 3 (halve the underweight rate among children under 5 by 2015) and dramatically reduce child hunger and undernutrition in a single generation.

In Mauritania, a working group of government, UN and international non-governmental organization staff, supported by a facilitator, developed a detailed nutrition action plan. The outcome has already been positive. Coordinated distribution of vitamin A and mebendazole (a deworming drug) in the south, for example, has reduced resource waste and duplication of efforts. Another positive outcome has been the launch of an improved referral and monitoring system for supplementary and therapeutic feeding.

The direct impact on nutritional status is shown by improvements in specific indicators. Preliminary results of data collected in 2008 indicate substantial improvements in household consumption of adequately iodized salt and in rates of exclusive breastfeeding between 2007 and 2008. There is optimism that the programmatic efforts made through REACH will ultimately lead to improved growth, survival and development for Mauritania's children.

The work in Mauritania has also led to the formation of a West African regional nutrition working group, developed to improve support to country teams and help mainstream the REACH approach. The working group assists in-country facilitators; provides tools, workshops and advice; and fosters advocacy, research and capacity-building in collaboration with such regional bodies as the Economic Community of West African States.

Sources: UNICEF, 'Report on implementation of the Ending Child Hunger and Undernutrition Initiative', E/ICEF/2008/11, Executive Board Annual Session 2008 (19 May 2008); and *Enquête rapide nationale sur la nutrition et survie de l'enfant en Mauritanie*, Government of Mauritania, Ministry of Health, and UNICEF, Nouakchott, December 2008.

8. THE WAY FORWARD

Clear and compelling evidence on the magnitude of undernutrition as well as its consequences is well documented. Clear evidence also exists concerning effective interventions to prevent undernutrition and the critical window of opportunity to deliver them – during a woman's pregnancy and before a child reaches age 2.

Without delay, these effective interventions need to be implemented at scale. Evidence of successful programmes in a number of countries – salt iodization, vitamin A supplementation, exclusive breastfeeding and community-based treatment of severe acute malnutrition – shows that this can be done rapidly and effectively, and the experiences gained in these programmes can be used as a guide. Effective health and water and sanitation programmes to prevent and treat infectious diseases must go hand in hand with implementation of the package of nutrition interventions.

To sustain improvement, underlying causes of undernutrition such as social norms, gender and equity issues must be addressed. An improvement in the status of women – including access to education and health care, a higher degree of decision-making power and gender equality – will contribute to marked and sustained improvements in child nutrition. Poverty, chronic and acute emergencies, and lack of access to resources often lead to food and nutrition insecurity, and in these situations, social protection schemes as well as programmes to enhance food production and household food and nutrition security must be expanded.

A global momentum is needed that will entail unified and compelling advocacy among governments, lead organizations and institutions. Enhanced advocacy and resources, in combination with strengthened collaboration and effective coordination at the international level, should be reflected at the country level, with clear national ownership and leadership.

For the sake of the survival, growth and development of millions of children and the overall development of many countries, we cannot afford to neglect this issue.

REFERENCES

1. Pelletier, David L., et al., 'Epidemiologic Evidence for a Potentiating Effect of Malnutrition on Child Mortality', *American Journal of Public Health,* vol. 83, no. 8, August 1993, pp. 1130–1133; and Habicht, Jean-Pierre, 'Malnutrition Kills Directly, Not Indirectly', *The Lancet*, vol. 371, no. 9626, 24–30 May 2008, pp. 1749–1750.

2. Black, Robert E., et al., 'Maternal and Child Undernutrition: Global and regional exposures and health consequences', *The Lancet*, vol. 371, no. 9608, 19 January 2008, pp. 243–260. Note that earlier estimates of more than 50 per cent of deaths being caused by undernutrition relate to the age group 6–59 months, whereas the latest estimate extends to all children under 5 years old.

3. Black, Robert E., et al., 'Maternal and Child Undernutrition: Global and regional exposures and health consequences', *The Lancet*, vol. 371, no. 9608, 19 January 2008, pp. 243–260.

4. Ibid.

5. Pelletier, David L., et al., 'Epidemiologic Evidence for a Potentiating Effect of Malnutrition on Child Mortality', *American Journal of Public Health,* vol. 83, no. 8, August 1993, pp. 1130–1133; and Habicht, Jean-Pierre, 'Malnutrition Kills Directly, Not Indirectly', *The Lancet,* vol. 371, no. 9626, 24–30 May 2008, pp. 1749–1750.

6. Black, Robert E., et al., 'Maternal and Child Undernutrition: Global and regional exposures and health consequences', *The Lancet,* vol. 371, no. 9608, 19 January 2008, pp. 243–260.

7. Jones, Gareth, et al., 'How many child deaths can we prevent this year?' *The Lancet*, vol. 362, no. 9377, 5 July 2003, pp. 65–71.

8. WHO Collaborative Study Team on the Role of Breastfeeding on the Prevention of Infant Mortality, 'Effect of Breastfeeding on Infant and Child Mortality Due to Infectious Diseases in Less Developed Countries: A pooled analysis', *The Lancet,* vol. 355, no. 9202, 2000, pp. 451–455.

9. Beaton. G. H., et al., 'Effectiveness of Vitamin A Supplementation in the Control of Young Child Morbidity and Mortality in Developing Countries', *Nutrition Policy Discussion Paper,* no. 13, United Nations System Standing Committee on Nutrition, Geneva, 1993, pp. 4–6.

10. Micronutrient Initiative, 'Investing in the Future: A united call to action on vitamin and mineral deficiencies – Global report 2009', Micronutrient Initiative, Ottawa, 2009, pp. 5–6.

11. Shrimpton, Roger, et al., 'Worldwide Timing of Growth Faltering: Implications for nutritional interventions,' *Pediatrics,* vol. 107, no. 5, May 2001, pp. 5–6.

12. Victora, Cesar G., et al., 'Maternal and Child Undernutrition: Consequences for adult health and human capital', *The Lancet,* vol. 371, no. 9609, 26 January 2008, pp. 340–357.

13. Bleichrodt, N., and M. Born, 'A Meta-analysis of Research into Iodine and Its Relationship to Cognitive Development', in *The Damaged Brain of Iodine Deficiency,* edited by John B. Stanbury, Cognizant Communication Corporation, New York, 1994, pp. 195–200.

14. Lozoff, Betsy, Elias Jimenez and Julia B. Smith, 'Double Burden of Iron Deficiency and Low Socio-Economic Status: A longitudinal analysis of cognitive test scores to 19 years', *Archives of Pediatric & Adolescent Medicine,* vol. 160, no. 11, November 2006, pp. 1108–1113.

15. Black, Robert E., et al., 'Maternal and Child Undernutrition: Global and regional exposures and health consequences', *The Lancet,* vol. 371, no. 9608, 19 January 2008, pp. 243–260.

16. Hunt, Joseph, M., 'Reversing Productivity Losses from Iron Deficiency: The economic case', *Journal of Nutrition,* vol. 132, 4 suppl., April 2002, pp. 794S–801S.

17. Victora, Cesar G., et al., 'Maternal and Child Undernutrition: Consequences for adult health and human capital', *The Lancet,* vol. 371, no. 9609, 26 January 2008, pp. 340–357.

18. Ibid.

19. Ibid.

20. Hoddinott, John, et al., 'Effect of a Nutrition Intervention during Early Childhood on Economic Productivity in Guatemalan Adults', *The Lancet,* vol. 371, 2 February 2008, pp. 411–416.

21. Republic of Honduras and ORC Macro, 'National Demographic and Health Survey, 2005–06', Macro International, Calverton, MD, December 2006.

22. World Health Organization, 'Global Prevalence of Vitamin A Deficiency in Populations at Risk 1995–2005: WHO global database on vitamin A deficiency', WHO, Geneva, 2009, pp. 10–11.

23. Benoist, Bruno de, et al., editors, 'Worldwide Prevalence of Anaemia 1993–2005: WHO global database on anaemia', World Health Organization and Centers for Disease Control and Prevention, Geneva and Atlanta, GA, 2008, p. 8.

24. Benoist, Bruno de, et al., 'Iodine Deficiency in 2007: Global progress since 2003', *Food and Nutrition Bulletin,* vol. 29, no. 3, 2008, pp. 195–202.

25. Edmond, Karen, et al., 'Delayed Breastfeeding Initiation Increases Risk of Neonatal Mortality', *Pediatrics,* vol. 117, no. 3, 1 March 2006, pp. e380–e386; and Mullany, Luke C., et al., 'Breastfeeding Patterns, Time to Initiation and Mortality Risk Among Newborns in Southern Nepal', *Journal of Nutrition,* vol. 138, March 2008, pp. 599–603.

26. Huffman, Sandra L., et al., 'Can Improvements in Breast-feeding Practices Reduce Neonatal Mortality in Developing Countries?', *Midwifery,* vol. 17, no. 2, June 2001, pp. 84–86.

27. Ramakrishnan, Usha, et al., 'Effects of Micronutrients on Growth of Children under 5 Years of Age: Meta-analyses of single and multiple nutrient interventions', *American Journal of Clinical Nutrition,* vol. 89, no. 1, January 2009, pp. 191–203.

28. UNICEF analysis of data from 109 rounds of vitamin A delivery in 55 countries in 2008 (internal database, 2008).

29. Flour Fortification Initiative, 'Map of Global Progress: Fortification status – March 2009', FFI, Atlanta, GA, <www.sph.emory.edu/wheatflour/globalmap.php>, accessed 25 September 2009.

30. Dewey, Kathryn G., et al., 'Systematic Review and Meta-Analysis of Home Fortification of Complementary Foods', *Maternal and Child Nutrition,* 2009, vol. 5, issue 4, pp. 283–321.

31. United Nations Children's Fund, 'Workshop Report on Scaling Up the Use of Multiple Micronutrient Powders to Improve the Quality of Complementary Foods for Young Children in Asia', UNICEF, 2009, p. 2.

32. Haddad, Lawrence, et al., 'Reducing Child Undernutrition: How far does income growth take us?', FCND *Discussion Paper,* no. 137, International Food Policy Research Institute, Washington, D.C., August 2002, p. 24.

33. Hunt, Joseph M., 'The Potential Impact of Reducing Global Malnutrition on Poverty Reduction and Economic Development', *Asia Pacific Journal of Clinical Nutrition,* vol.14, CD Supplement, pp. 10–38.

34. Jolly, Richard, 'Nutrition', Our Planet, United Nations Environment Programme, 1996, <www.ourplanet.com/imgversn/122/jolly.html>, accessed 25 September 2009.

35 UNICEF analysis of Demographic and Health Survey data from the Plurinational State of Bolivia (2003) and Peru (2004–2006).

36 Dancer, Diane, Anu Rammohan and Murray D. Smith, 'Infant Mortality and Child Nutrition in Bangladesh', *Health Economics*, vol. 17, no. 9, September 2008, pp. 1015–1035.

37 Wamani, Henry, et al., 'Boys Are More Stunted than Girls in Sub-Saharan Africa: A meta-analysis of 16 demographic and health surveys', *BMC Pediatrics*, vol. 7, no. 17, 10 April 2007.

38 Cleland, John G., and Jeroen K. van Ginneken, 'Maternal Education and Child Survival in Developing Countries: The search for pathways of influence', *Social Science and Medicine*, vol. 27, no. 12, 1988, pp. 1357–1368.

39 Liaqat, Perveen, et al., 'Association between Complementary Feeding Practice and Mothers Education Status in Islamabad', *Journal of Human Nutrition and Dietetics*, vol. 20, no. 4, 17 July 2007, pp. 340–344.

40 Shroff, M., et al., 'Maternal Autonomy is Inversely Related to Child Stunting in Andhra Pradesh, India', *Maternal and Child Nutrition*, vol. 5, no. 1, 1 January 2009, pp. 64–74.

41 World Health Organization, United Nations Children's Fund, Academy for Educational Development and United States Agency for Development, 'Learning from Large-Scale Community Based Programmes to Improve Breastfeeding Practices: Report of ten-country case study', WHO, Geneva, 2008, pp. 7–8, 10–12, 21.

42 United Nations Children's Fund, 'Annual report of the Executive Director: Progress and achievements against the medium-term strategic plan', Executive Board, Annual session 2009, 8–10 June 2009, E/ICEF/2009/9*, p. 6.

43 UNICEF, 'A Supply Chain Analysis of Ready-to-use Therapeutic Foods for the Horn of Africa: The Nutrition Articulation Project. A Study', May 2009, pp. i and 12.

44 Horton, Sue, Harold Alderman and Juan A. Rivera, 'Copenhagen Consensus 2008 Challenge Paper: Hunger and malnutrition', Copenhagen Consensus Center, Frederiksberg, Denmark, May 2008, p. 32.

45 Lechtig, A., et al., 'Decreasing stunting, anemia, and vitamin A deficiency in Peru: Results of The Good Start in Life Program', *Food and Nutrition Bulletin*, vol. 30, no. 1, March 2009, p. 37.

46 Boston Consulting Group, 'REACH: Successful practice compilation and country pilots, High-level cost estimates for REACH-promoted interventions' (presentation), August 2008.

Notes on the maps

For the maps on page 15 ('195 million children in the developing world are stunted' and 'Stunting prevalence worldwide'), page 18 ('Underweight prevalence worldwide') and page 21 ('Wasting prevalence'), estimates are calculated according to the WHO Child Growth Standards, except in cases where data are only available according to the previously used NCHS/WHO reference population. Estimates for 96 countries are from surveys conducted in 2003 or later.

For the map on page 19 ('63 countries are on track to meet the MDG 1 target'), estimates are calculated according to the NCHS/WHO reference population.

For the map on page 24 ('Exclusive breastfeeding rates'), estimates for 108 countries are from surveys conducted in 2003 or later.

For more information on countries with estimates calculated according to the NCHS/WHO reference population or countries with surveys before 2003, please refer to data notes on page 116.

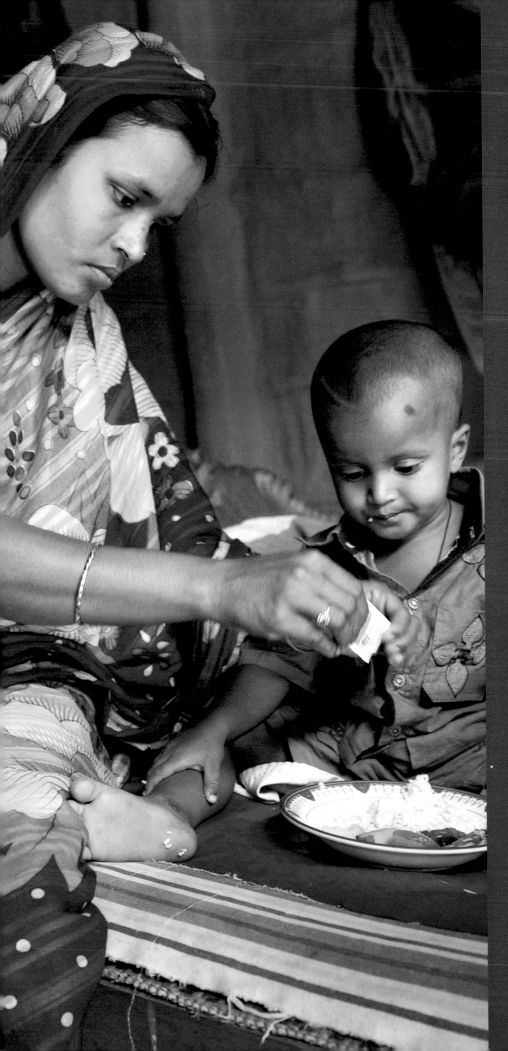

NUTRITION PROFILES:

**24 countries
with the largest
burden of stunting**

AFGHANISTAN

DEMOGRAPHICS

Total population (000)	27,208	(2008)
Total under-five population (000)	4,907	(2008)
Total number of births (000)	1,269	(2008)
Under-five mortality rate (per 1,000 live births)	257	(2008)
Total number of under-five deaths (000)	311	(2008)
Infant mortality rate (per 1,000 live births)	165	(2008)
Neonatal mortality rate (per 1,000 live births)	60	(2004)
HIV prevalence rate (15–49 years, %)	-	
Population below international poverty line of US$1.25 per day (%)	-	

Under-five mortality rate
Deaths per 1,000 live births

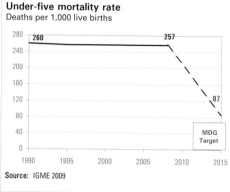

Source: IGME 2009

Causes of under-five deaths, 2004

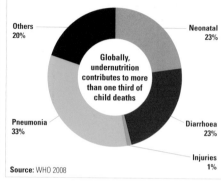

Globally, undernutrition contributes to more than one third of child deaths

- Others 20%
- Neonatal 23%
- Diarrhoea 23%
- Injuries 1%
- Pneumonia 33%

Source: WHO 2008

NUTRITIONAL STATUS

Burden of undernutrition (2008)
WHO Child Growth Standards

Stunted (under-fives, 000):	2,910	Underweight (under-fives, 000):	1,614
Share of developing world stunting burden (%):	1.5	Wasted (under-fives, 000):	422
Stunting country rank:	11	Severely wasted (under-fives, 000):	172

Current nutritional status
Percentage of children < 5 years old suffering from:

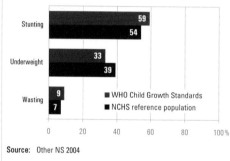

- Stunting: 59 (WHO Child Growth Standards), 54 (NCHS reference population)
- Underweight: 33 (WHO Child Growth Standards), 39 (NCHS reference population)
- Wasting: 9 (WHO Child Growth Standards), 7 (NCHS reference population)

Source: Other NS 2004

Stunting trends
Percentage of children < 5 years old stunted NCHS reference population

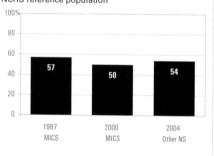

1997 MICS	2000 MICS	2004 Other NS
57	50	54

Underweight trends
Percentage of children < 5 years old underweight NCHS reference population

On track towards MDG1

1997 MICS	2000 MICS	2004 Other NS
49	47	39

INFANT AND YOUNG CHILD FEEDING

Child feeding practices, by age

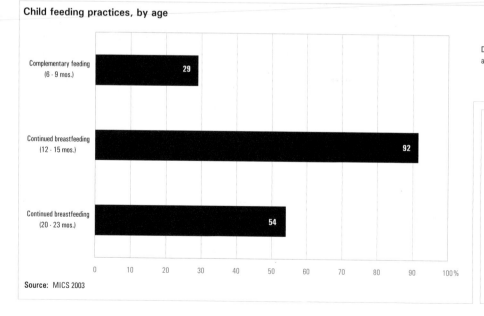

- Complementary feeding (6 - 9 mos.): 29
- Continued breastfeeding (12 - 15 mos.): 92
- Continued breastfeeding (20 - 23 mos.): 54

Source: MICS 2003

Data not available to produce infant feeding practices area graph

Exclusive breastfeeding
Percentage of infants < 6 months old exclusively breastfed

No data

MICRONUTRIENTS

Vitamin A supplementation
Percentage of children 6-59 months old receiving two doses of vitamin A during calendar year

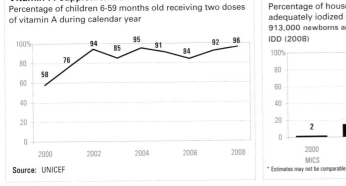

Source: UNICEF

Iodized salt consumption trends*
Percentage of households consuming adequately iodized salt
913,000 newborns are unprotected against IDD (2008)

* Estimates may not be comparable.

Anaemia
Prevalence of anaemia among selected population

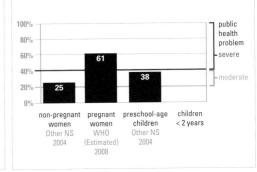

ESSENTIAL NUTRITION INTERVENTIONS DURING THE LIFE CYCLE

Pregnancy	Birth	0-5 months	6-23 months	24-59 months

Use of iron-folic acid supplements	-	Early initiation of breastfeeding (within 1 hour of birth)	-	International Code of Marketing of Breastmilk Substitutes — Partial
				Maternity protection in accordance with ILO Convention 183 — No
Household consumption of adequately iodized salt	28%	Infants not weighed at birth	-	Exclusive breastfeeding (<6 months) —
				Timely introduction of complementary foods (with continued breastfeeding) — 29%
				Continued breastfeeding at two years — 54%

To increase children's chances of survival, improve development and prevent stunting, nutrition interventions need to be delivered during the mother's pregnancy and the first two years of the child's life.

Full coverage of vitamin A supplementation	96%
National guidelines for management of severe acute malnutrition incorporating the community-based approach	Yes
Policy on new ORS formula and zinc for management of diarrhoea	Partial
Policy on community treatment of pneumonia with antibiotics	Yes

MATERNAL NUTRITION/HEALTH

Maternal mortality ratio, adjusted (per 100,000 live births)	1,800	(2005)
Maternal mortality ratio, reported (per 100,000 live births)	1,600	(1999-2002)
Total number of maternal deaths	26,000	(2005)
Lifetime risk of maternal death (1 in :)	8	(2005)
Women with low BMI (<18.5 kg/m², %)	-	-
Anaemia, non-pregnant women (<120 g/l, %)	25	(2004)
Antenatal care (at least one visit, %)	16	(2003)
Antenatal care (at least four visits, %)	-	-
Skilled attendant at birth (%)	14	(2003)
Low birthweight (<2,500 grams, %)	-	-
Primary school net enrolment or attendance ratio (% female, % male)	46, 74	(2007)
Gender parity index (primary school net enrolment or attendance ratio)	0.62	(2007)

WATER AND SANITATION

Drinking water coverage
Percentage of population by type of drinking water source, 2006

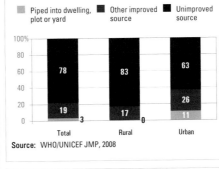

Source: WHO/UNICEF JMP, 2008

Sanitation coverage
Percentage of population by type of sanitation facility, 2006

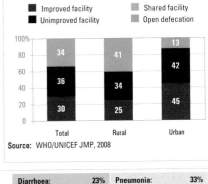

Source: WHO/UNICEF JMP, 2008

Under-five deaths (post-neonatal) caused by:	Diarrhoea:	23%	Pneumonia:	33%

DISPARITIES IN NUTRITION

Indicator	Gender			Residence			Wealth quintile						Source
	Male	Female	Ratio of male to female	Urban	Rural	Ratio of urban to rural	Poorest	Second	Middle	Fourth	Richest	Ratio of richest to poorest	
Stunting prevalence (WHO Child Growth Standards, %)	60	59	1.0	-	-	-	-	-	-	-	-	-	Other NS 2004
Underweight prevalence (WHO Child Growth Standards, %)	33	33	1.0	-	-	-	-	-	-	-	-	-	Other NS 2004
Wasting prevalence (WHO Child Growth Standards, %)	8	9	0.9	-	-	-	-	-	-	-	-	-	Other NS 2004
Infants not weighed at birth (%)	-	-	-	-	-	-	-	-	-	-	-	-	-
Early initiation of breastfeeding (%)	-	-	-	-	-	-	-	-	-	-	-	-	-
Women with low BMI (<18.5 kg/m², %)	-	-	-	-	-	-	-	-	-	-	-	-	-

BANGLADESH

Total population (000)	160,000	(2008)
Total under-five population (000)	16,710	(2008)
Total number of births (000)	3,430	(2008)
Under-five mortality rate (per 1,000 live births)	54	(2008)
Total number of under-five deaths (000)	183	(2008)
Infant mortality rate (per 1,000 live births)	43	(2008)
Neonatal mortality rate (per 1,000 live births)	36	(2004)
HIV prevalence rate (15–49 years, %)	-	
Population below international poverty line of US$1.25 per day (%)	50	(2005)

Under-five mortality rate
Deaths per 1,000 live births

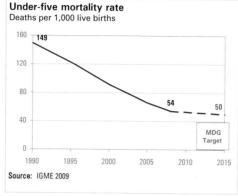

Source: IGME 2009

Causes of under-five deaths, 2004

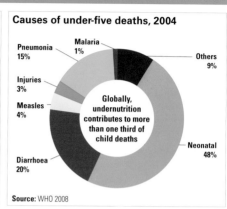

Globally, undernutrition contributes to more than one third of child deaths

Pneumonia 15%
Malaria 1%
Others 9%
Injuries 3%
Measles 4%
Diarrhoea 20%
Neonatal 48%

Source: WHO 2008

NUTRITIONAL STATUS

Burden of undernutrition (2008)
WHO Child Growth Standards

Stunted (under-fives, 000):	7,219	Underweight (under-fives, 000):	6,851
Share of developing world stunting burden (%):	3.7	Wasted (under-fives, 000):	2,908
Stunting country rank:	6	Severely wasted (under-fives, 000):	485

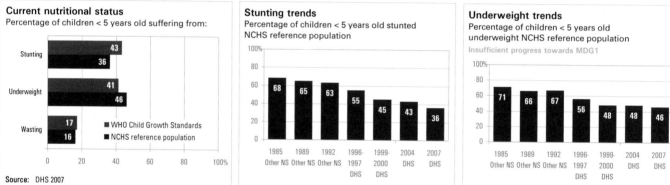

Current nutritional status
Percentage of children < 5 years old suffering from:

Stunting 43 / 36
Underweight 41 / 46
Wasting 17 / 16

■ WHO Child Growth Standards
■ NCHS reference population

Source: DHS 2007

Stunting trends
Percentage of children < 5 years old stunted
NCHS reference population

1985 Other NS: 68
1989 Other NS: 65
1992 Other NS: 63
1996-1997 DHS: 55
1999-2000 DHS: 45
2004 DHS: 43
2007 DHS: 36

Underweight trends
Percentage of children < 5 years old
underweight NCHS reference population
Insufficient progress towards MDG1

1985 Other NS: 71
1989 Other NS: 66
1992 Other NS: 67
1996-1997 DHS: 56
1999-2000 DHS: 48
2004 DHS: 48
2007 DHS: 46

INFANT AND YOUNG CHILD FEEDING

Infant feeding practices, by age

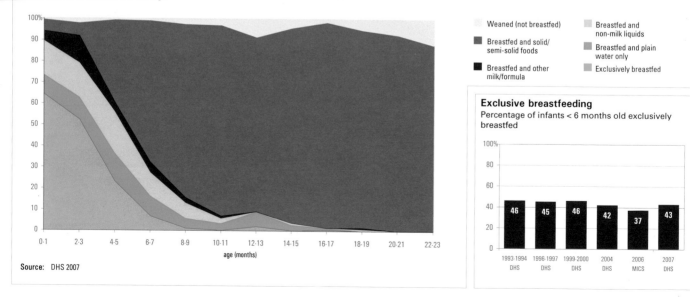

age (months)

□ Weaned (not breastfed)
■ Breastfed and solid/semi-solid foods
■ Breastfed and other milk/formula
■ Breastfed and non-milk liquids
■ Breastfed and plain water only
■ Exclusively breastfed

Source: DHS 2007

Exclusive breastfeeding
Percentage of infants < 6 months old exclusively breastfed

1993-1994 DHS: 46
1996-1997 DHS: 45
1999-2000 DHS: 46
2004 DHS: 42
2006 MICS: 37
2007 DHS: 43

MICRONUTRIENTS

Vitamin A supplementation
Percentage of children 6-59 months old receiving two doses of vitamin A during calendar year

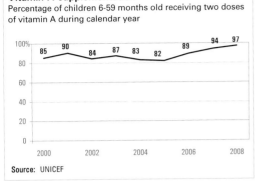

Values: 85, 90, 84, 87, 83, 82, 89, 94, 97 (2000–2008)

Source: UNICEF

Iodized salt consumption trends*
Percentage of households consuming adequately iodized salt
538,000 newborns are unprotected against IDD (2008)

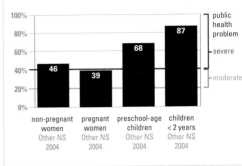

1995 MICS	2000 MICS	2003 MICS	2006 MICS
44	70	70	84

* Estimates may not be comparable.

Anaemia
Prevalence of anaemia among selected population

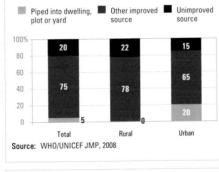

non-pregnant women Other NS 2004	pregnant women Other NS 2004	preschool-age children Other NS 2004	children < 2 years Other NS 2004
46	39	68	87

public health problem / severe / moderate

ESSENTIAL NUTRITION INTERVENTIONS DURING THE LIFE CYCLE

| Pregnancy | Birth | 0-5 months | 6-23 months | 24-59 months |

Use of iron-folic acid supplements	-	Early initiation of breastfeeding (within 1 hour of birth)	43%	International Code of Marketing of Breastmilk Substitutes	Partial

| | | | | Maternity protection in accordance with ILO Convention 183 | No |

| Household consumption of adequately iodized salt | 84% | Infants not weighed at birth | 85% | Exclusive breastfeeding (<6 months) | 43% | Timely introduction of complementary foods (with continued breastfeeding) | 74% |

| | | | | | | Continued breastfeeding at two years | 91% |

To increase children's chances of survival, improve development and prevent stunting, nutrition interventions need to be delivered during the mother's pregnancy and the first two years of the child's life.

Full coverage of vitamin A supplementation	97%
National guidelines for management of severe acute malnutrition incorporating the community-based approach	No
Policy on new ORS formula and zinc for management of diarrhoea	Yes
Policy on community treatment of pneumonia with antibiotics	Partial

MATERNAL NUTRITION/HEALTH

Maternal mortality ratio, adjusted (per 100,000 live births)	570	(2005)
Maternal mortality ratio, reported (per 100,000 live births)	350	(2007)
Total number of maternal deaths	21,000	(2005)
Lifetime risk of maternal death (1 in :)	51	(2005)
Women with low BMI (<18.5 kg/m², %)	30	(2007)
Anaemia, non-pregnant women (<120 g/l, %)	46	(2004)
Antenatal care (at least one visit, %)	51	(2007)
Antenatal care (at least four visits, %)	21	(2007)
Skilled attendant at birth (%)	18	(2007)
Low birthweight (<2,500 grams, %)	22	(2006)
Primary school net enrolment or attendance ratio (% female, % male)	84, 79	(2006)
Gender parity index (primary school net enrolment or attendance ratio)	1.06	(2006)

WATER AND SANITATION

Drinking water coverage
Percentage of population by type of drinking water source, 2006

Piped into dwelling, plot or yard / Other improved source / Unimproved source

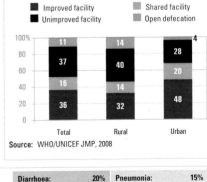

	Total	Rural	Urban
Unimproved source	20	22	15
Other improved source	75	78	65
Piped into dwelling, plot or yard	5	0	20

Source: WHO/UNICEF JMP, 2008

Sanitation coverage
Percentage of population by type of sanitation facility, 2006

Improved facility / Shared facility / Unimproved facility / Open defecation

	Total	Rural	Urban
Open defecation	11	14	4
Unimproved facility	37	40	28
Shared facility	16	14	20
Improved facility	36	32	48

Source: WHO/UNICEF JMP, 2008

Under-five deaths (post-neonatal) caused by: Diarrhoea: 20% | Pneumonia: 15%

DISPARITIES IN NUTRITION

Indicator	Gender			Residence			Wealth quintile						Source
	Male	Female	Ratio of male to female	Urban	Rural	Ratio of urban to rural	Poorest	Second	Middle	Fourth	Richest	Ratio of richest to poorest	
Stunting prevalence (WHO Child Growth Standards, %)	44	43	1.0	36	45	0.8	54	51	42	39	26	0.5	DHS 2007
Underweight prevalence (WHO Child Growth Standards, %)	40	42	1.0	33	43	0.8	51	46	41	38	26	0.5	DHS 2007
Wasting prevalence (WHO Child Growth Standards, %)	18	17	1.1	14	18	0.8	21	18	17	18	13	0.6	DHS 2007
Infants not weighed at birth (%)	-	-	-	73	89	0.8	92	93	89	84	58	0.6	MICS 2006
Early initiation of breastfeeding (%)	44	42	1.0	41	43	1.0	43	43	43	44	40	0.9	DHS 2007
Women with low BMI (<18.5 kg/m², %)	-	30	-	20	33	0.6	43	35	33	25	13	0.3	DHS 2007

CHINA

DEMOGRAPHICS

Total population (000)	1,337,411	(2008)
Total under-five population (000)	86,881	(2008)
Total number of births (000)	18,134	(2008)
Under-five mortality rate (per 1,000 live births)	21	(2008)
Total number of under-five deaths (000)	365	(2008)
Infant mortality rate (per 1,000 live births)	18	(2008)
Neonatal mortality rate (per 1,000 live births)	18	(2004)
HIV prevalence rate (15–49 years, %)	0.1	(2007)
Population below international poverty line of US$1.25 per day (%)	16	(2005)

Under-five mortality rate
Deaths per 1,000 live births

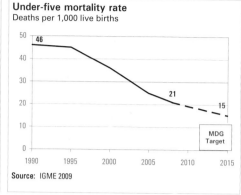

Source: IGME 2009

Causes of under-five deaths, 2004

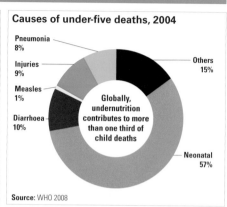

Pneumonia 8%
Injuries 9%
Measles 1%
Diarrhoea 10%
Others 15%
Neonatal 57%

Globally, undernutrition contributes to more than one third of child deaths

Source: WHO 2008

NUTRITIONAL STATUS

Burden of undernutrition (2008)
WHO Child Growth Standards

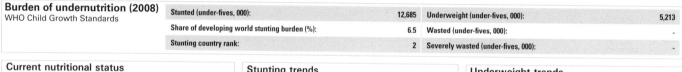

Stunted (under-fives, 000):	12,685	Underweight (under-fives, 000):	5,213
Share of developing world stunting burden (%):	6.5	Wasted (under-fives, 000):	-
Stunting country rank:	2	Severely wasted (under-fives, 000):	-

Current nutritional status
Percentage of children < 5 years old suffering from:

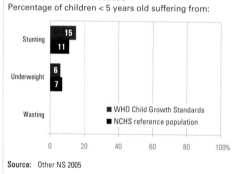

Stunting 15 / 11
Underweight 6 / 7
Wasting

■ WHO Child Growth Standards
■ NCHS reference population

Source: Other NS 2005

Stunting trends
Percentage of children < 5 years old stunted
NCHS reference population

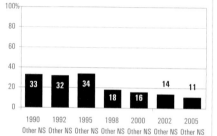

1990	1992	1995	1998	2000	2002	2005
Other NS	Other NS	Other NS	Other NS	Other NS	Other NS	Other NS
33	32	34	18	16	14	11

Underweight trends
Percentage of children < 5 years old
underweight NCHS reference population
On track towards MDG1

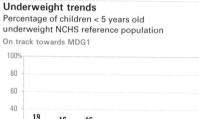

1990	1992	1995	1998	2000	2002	2005
Other NS	Other NS	Other NS	Other NS	Other NS	Other NS	Other NS
19	16	16	10	10	8	7

INFANT AND YOUNG CHILD FEEDING

Child feeding practices, by age

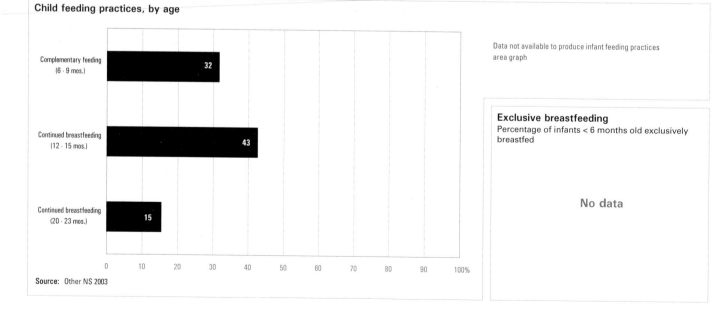

Complementary feeding (6 - 9 mos.) 32
Continued breastfeeding (12 - 15 mos.) 43
Continued breastfeeding (20 - 23 mos.) 15

Source: Other NS 2003

Data not available to produce infant feeding practices area graph

Exclusive breastfeeding
Percentage of infants < 6 months old exclusively breastfed

No data

MICRONUTRIENTS

Vitamin A supplementation
Percentage of children 6-59 months old receiving two doses of vitamin A during calendar year

Subnational Programme

Iodized salt consumption trends*
Percentage of households consuming adequately iodized salt
943,000 newborns are unprotected against IDD (2008)

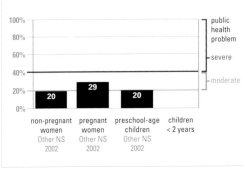

1995	2002	2008
60	93	95
Other NS	Other NS	Other NS

* Estimates may not be comparable.

Anaemia
Prevalence of anaemia among selected population

non-pregnant women Other NS 2002	pregnant women Other NS 2002	preschool-age children Other NS 2002	children < 2 years
20	29	20	

public health problem
— severe
— moderate

ESSENTIAL NUTRITION INTERVENTIONS DURING THE LIFE CYCLE

Pregnancy >	Birth >	0-5 months >	6-23 months >	24-59 months >

Use of iron-folic acid supplements	-	Early initiation of breastfeeding (within 1 hour of birth)	-

International Code of Marketing of Breastmilk Substitutes	Partial
Maternity protection in accordance with ILO Convention 183	No

Household consumption of adequately iodized salt	95%	Infants not weighed at birth	-

Exclusive breastfeeding (<6 months)	-

Timely introduction of complementary foods (with continued breastfeeding)	32%
Continued breastfeeding at two years	15%

To increase children's chances of survival, improve development and prevent stunting, nutrition interventions need to be delivered during the mother's pregnancy and the first two years of the child's life.

Full coverage of vitamin A supplementation	SP*
National guidelines for management of severe acute malnutrition incorporating the community-based approach	NA*
Policy on new ORS formula and zinc for management of diarrhoea	Partial
Policy on community treatment of pneumonia with antibiotics	Partial

*SP: Subnational programme
*NA: Not applicable

MATERNAL NUTRITION/HEALTH

Maternal mortality ratio, adjusted (per 100,000 live births)	45	(2005)
Maternal mortality ratio, reported (per 100,000 live births)	37	(2007)
Total number of maternal deaths	7,800	(2005)
Lifetime risk of maternal death (1 in :)	1,300	(2005)
Women with low BMI (<18.5 kg/m², %)	-	-
Anaemia, non-pregnant women (<120 g/l, %)	20	(2002)
Antenatal care (at least one visit, %)	91	(2007)
Antenatal care (at least four visits, %)	-	-
Skilled attendant at birth (%)	98	(2007)
Low birthweight (<2,500 grams, %)	4	(1999-2003)
Primary school net enrolment or attendance ratio (% female, % male)	100, 100	(2007)
Gender parity index (primary school net enrolment or attendance ratio)	1.00	(2007)

WATER AND SANITATION

Drinking water coverage
Percentage of population by type of drinking water source, 2006

- Piped into dwelling, plot or yard
- Other improved source
- Unimproved source

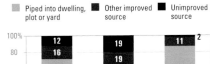

	Total	Rural	Urban
Unimproved source	12	19	11 (2)
Other improved	16	19	
Piped	72	62	87

Source: WHO/UNICEF JMP, 2008

Sanitation coverage
Percentage of population by type of sanitation facility, 2006

- Improved facility
- Unimproved facility
- Shared facility
- Open defecation

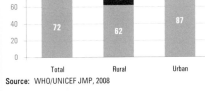

	Total	Rural	Urban
	25 (3)	38 (2)	7/15 (4)
	7	1	
Improved	65	59	74

Source: WHO/UNICEF JMP, 2008

Under-five deaths (post-neonatal) caused by: Diarrhoea: 10% Pneumonia: 8%

DISPARITIES IN NUTRITION

Indicator	Gender			Residence			Wealth quintile						Source
	Male	Female	Ratio of male to female	Urban	Rural	Ratio of urban to rural	Poorest	Second	Middle	Fourth	Richest	Ratio of richest to poorest	
Stunting prevalence (WHO Child Growth Standards, %)	23	21	1.1	9	26	0.3	-	-	-	-	-	-	Other NS 2002
Underweight prevalence (WHO Child Growth Standards, %)	7	7	1.0	3	8	0.4	-	-	-	-	-	-	Other NS 2002
Wasting prevalence (WHO Child Growth Standards, %)	3	3	1.0	2	3	0.7	-	-	-	-	-	-	Other NS 2002
Infants not weighed at birth (%)	-	-	-	-	-	-	-	-	-	-	-	-	-
Early initiation of breastfeeding (%)	-	-	-	-	-	-	-	-	-	-	-	-	-
Women with low BMI (<18.5 kg/m², %)	-	-	-	-	-	-	-	-	-	-	-	-	-

DEMOGRAPHICS

Total population (000)	64,257	(2008)
Total under-five population (000)	11,829	(2008)
Total number of births (000)	2,886	(2008)
Under-five mortality rate (per 1,000 live births)	199	(2008)
Total number of under-five deaths (000)	554	(2008)
Infant mortality rate (per 1,000 live births)	126	(2008)
Neonatal mortality rate (per 1,000 live births)	47	(2004)
HIV prevalence rate (15–49 years, %)	-	
Population below international poverty line of US$1.25 per day (%)	59	(2005-2006)

Under-five mortality rate
Deaths per 1,000 live births

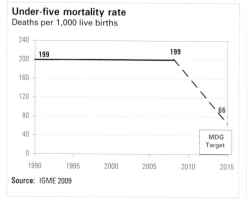

Source: IGME 2009

Causes of under-five deaths, 2004

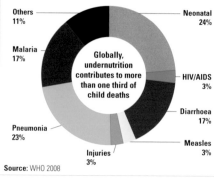

Others 11%
Neonatal 24%
Malaria 17%
HIV/AIDS 3%
Diarrhoea 17%
Pneumonia 23%
Measles 3%
Injuries 3%

Globally, undernutrition contributes to more than one third of child deaths

Source: WHO 2008

NUTRITIONAL STATUS

Burden of undernutrition (2008)
WHO Child Growth Standards

Stunted (under-fives, 000):	5,382	Underweight (under-fives, 000):	2,969
Share of developing world stunting burden (%):	2.8	Wasted (under-fives, 000):	1,183
Stunting country rank:	8	Severely wasted (under-fives, 000):	509

Current nutritional status
Percentage of children < 5 years old suffering from:

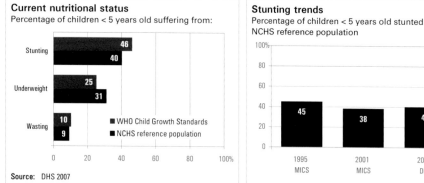

Stunting 46 / 40
Underweight 25 / 31
Wasting 10 / 9

■ WHO Child Growth Standards
■ NCHS reference population

Source: DHS 2007

Stunting trends
Percentage of children < 5 years old stunted NCHS reference population

1995 MICS: 45
2001 MICS: 38
2007 DHS: 40

Underweight trends
Percentage of children < 5 years old underweight NCHS reference population

Insufficient progress towards MDG1

1995 MICS: 34
2001 MICS: 31
2007 DHS: 31

INFANT AND YOUNG CHILD FEEDING

Infant feeding practices, by age

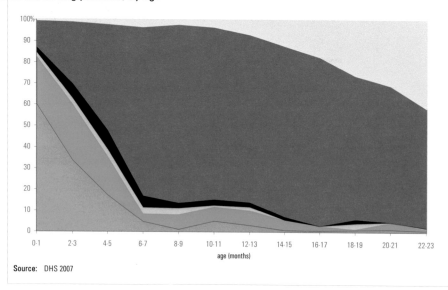

age (months)

Source: DHS 2007

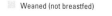

☐ Weaned (not breastfed)
■ Breastfed and solid/semi-solid foods
■ Breastfed and other milk/formula
☐ Breastfed and non-milk liquids
■ Breastfed and plain water only
■ Exclusively breastfed

Exclusive breastfeeding
Percentage of infants < 6 months old exclusively breastfed

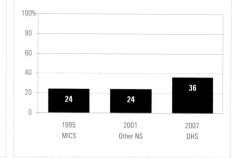

1995 MICS: 24
2001 Other NS: 24
2007 DHS: 36

MICRONUTRIENTS

Vitamin A supplementation
Percentage of children 6-59 months old receiving two doses of vitamin A during calendar year

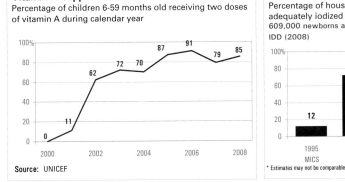

Source: UNICEF

Iodized salt consumption trends*
Percentage of households consuming adequately iodized salt
609,000 newborns are unprotected against IDD (2008)

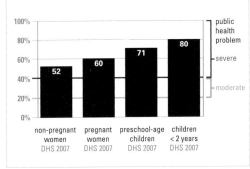

1995 MICS — 12
2001 MICS — 72
2007 DHS — 79

* Estimates may not be comparable.

Anaemia
Prevalence of anaemia among selected population

non-pregnant women DHS 2007 — 52
pregnant women DHS 2007 — 60
preschool-age children DHS 2007 — 71
children < 2 years DHS 2007 — 80

public health problem / severe / moderate

ESSENTIAL NUTRITION INTERVENTIONS DURING THE LIFE CYCLE

Pregnancy	Birth	0-5 months	6-23 months	24-59 months

Use of iron-folic acid supplements	2%	Early initiation of breastfeeding (within 1 hour of birth)	48%
Household consumption of adequately iodized salt	79%	Infants not weighed at birth	32%

International Code of Marketing of Breastmilk Substitutes	Yes
Maternity protection in accordance with ILO Convention 183	No

Exclusive breastfeeding (<6 months)	36%

Timely introduction of complementary foods (with continued breastfeeding)	82%
Continued breastfeeding at two years	64%
Full coverage of vitamin A supplementation	85%
National guidelines for management of severe acute malnutrition incorporating the community-based approach	Yes
Policy on new ORS formula and zinc for management of diarrhoea	Yes
Policy on community treatment of pneumonia with antibiotics	Yes

To increase children's chances of survival, improve development and prevent stunting, nutrition interventions need to be delivered during the mother's pregnancy and the first two years of the child's life.

MATERNAL NUTRITION/HEALTH

Maternal mortality ratio, adjusted (per 100,000 live births)	1,100	(2005)
Maternal mortality ratio, reported (per 100,000 live births)	550	(2004-2007)
Total number of maternal deaths	32,000	(2005)
Lifetime risk of maternal death (1 in :)	13	(2005)
Women with low BMI (<18.5 kg/m², %)	19	(2007)
Anaemia, non-pregnant women (<120 g/l, %)	52	(2007)
Antenatal care (at least one visit, %)	85	(2007)
Antenatal care (at least four visits, %)	47	(2007)
Skilled attendant at birth (%)	74	(2007)
Low birthweight (<2,500 grams, %)	12	(2001)
Primary school net enrolment or attendance ratio (% female, % male)	59, 63	(2007)
Gender parity index (primary school net enrolment or attendance ratio)	0.94	(2007)

WATER AND SANITATION

Drinking water coverage
Percentage of population by type of drinking water source, 2006

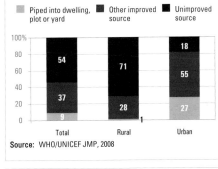

Piped into dwelling, plot or yard / Other improved source / Unimproved source

Total — 54, 37, 9
Rural — 71, 28, 1
Urban — 18, 55, 27

Source: WHO/UNICEF JMP, 2008

Sanitation coverage
Percentage of population by type of sanitation facility, 2006

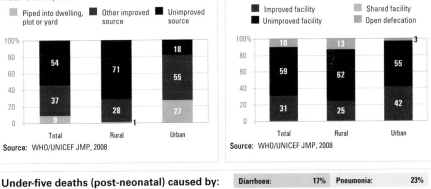

Improved facility / Shared facility / Unimproved facility / Open defecation

Total — 10, 59, 31
Rural — 13, 62, 25
Urban — 3, 55, 42

Source: WHO/UNICEF JMP, 2008

Under-five deaths (post-neonatal) caused by: Diarrhoea: 17% Pneumonia: 23%

DISPARITIES IN NUTRITION

Indicator	Gender			Residence			Wealth quintile						Source
	Male	Female	Ratio of male to female	Urban	Rural	Ratio of urban to rural	Poorest	Second	Middle	Fourth	Richest	Ratio of richest to poorest	
Stunting prevalence (WHO Child Growth Standards, %)	48	43	1.1	37	52	0.7	47	49	53	48	26	0.6	DHS 2007
Underweight prevalence (WHO Child Growth Standards, %)	28	23	1.2	19	29	0.7	27	29	28	25	15	0.6	DHS 2007
Wasting prevalence (WHO Child Growth Standards, %)	11	9	1.2	10	10	1.0	10	12	9	10	9	0.9	DHS 2007
Infants not weighed at birth (%)	-	-	-	11	46	0.2	53	47	33	17	3	0.1	DHS 2007
Early initiation of breastfeeding (%)	47	49	1.0	47	49	1.0	45	48	51	51	45	1.0	DHS 2007
Women with low BMI (<18.5 kg/m², %)	-	19	-	16	21	0.8	23	20	21	15	15	0.7	DHS 2007

EGYPT

DEMOGRAPHICS

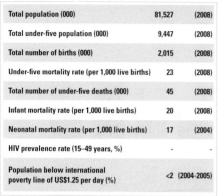

Total population (000)	81,527	(2008)
Total under-five population (000)	9,447	(2008)
Total number of births (000)	2,015	(2008)
Under-five mortality rate (per 1,000 live births)	23	(2008)
Total number of under-five deaths (000)	45	(2008)
Infant mortality rate (per 1,000 live births)	20	(2008)
Neonatal mortality rate (per 1,000 live births)	17	(2004)
HIV prevalence rate (15–49 years, %)	-	-
Population below international poverty line of US$1.25 per day (%)	<2	(2004-2005)

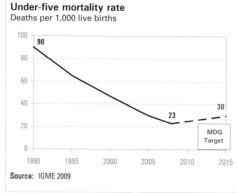

Under-five mortality rate
Deaths per 1,000 live births

Source: IGME 2009

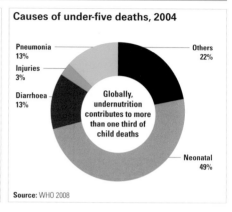

Causes of under-five deaths, 2004

Pneumonia 13%
Injuries 3%
Diarrhoea 13%
Others 22%
Neonatal 49%

Globally, undernutrition contributes to more than one third of child deaths

Source: WHO 2008

NUTRITIONAL STATUS

Burden of undernutrition (2008)
WHO Child Growth Standards

Stunted (under-fives, 000):	2,730	Underweight (under-fives, 000):	567
Share of developing world stunting burden (%):	1.4	Wasted (under-fives, 000):	680
Stunting country rank:	12	Severely wasted (under-fives, 000):	302

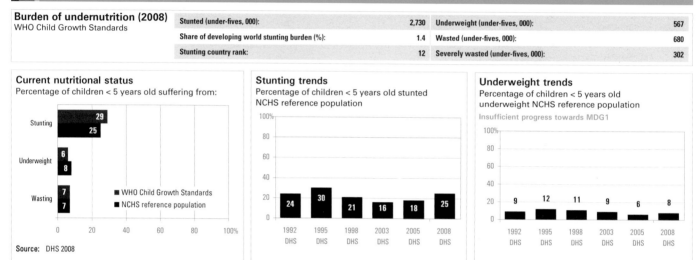

Current nutritional status
Percentage of children < 5 years old suffering from:

- Stunting: 29 / 25
- Underweight: 6 / 8
- Wasting: 7 / 7

■ WHO Child Growth Standards
■ NCHS reference population

Source: DHS 2008

Stunting trends
Percentage of children < 5 years old stunted
NCHS reference population

1992 DHS	1995 DHS	1998 DHS	2003 DHS	2005 DHS	2008 DHS
24	30	21	16	18	25

Underweight trends
Percentage of children < 5 years old
underweight NCHS reference population
Insufficient progress towards MDG1

1992 DHS	1995 DHS	1998 DHS	2003 DHS	2005 DHS	2008 DHS
9	12	11	9	6	8

INFANT AND YOUNG CHILD FEEDING

Infant feeding practices, by age

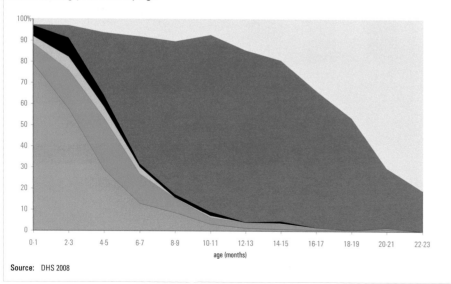

age (months)

Source: DHS 2008

- Weaned (not breastfed)
- Breastfed and solid/semi-solid foods
- Breastfed and other milk/formula
- Breastfed and non-milk liquids
- Breastfed and plain water only
- Exclusively breastfed

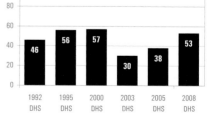

Exclusive breastfeeding
Percentage of infants < 6 months old exclusively breastfed

1992 DHS	1995 DHS	2000 DHS	2003 DHS	2005 DHS	2008 DHS
46	56	57	30	38	53

MICRONUTRIENTS

Vitamin A supplementation
Percentage of children 6-59 months old receiving two doses of vitamin A during calendar year

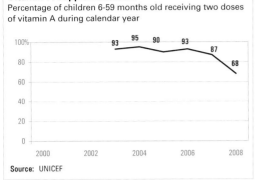

Source: UNICEF

Iodized salt consumption trends*
Percentage of households consuming adequately iodized salt
429,000 newborns are unprotected against IDD (2008)

2000 DHS	2003 DHS	2008 DHS
28	56	79

* Estimates may not be comparable.

Anaemia
Prevalence of anaemia among selected population

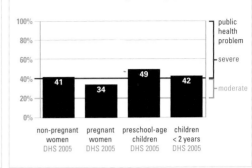

non-pregnant women DHS 2005	pregnant women DHS 2005	preschool-age children DHS 2005	children < 2 years DHS 2005
41	34	49	42

ESSENTIAL NUTRITION INTERVENTIONS DURING THE LIFE CYCLE

Pregnancy	Birth	0-5 months	6-23 months	24-59 months

| Use of iron-folic acid supplements | 14% |
| Household consumption of adequately iodized salt | 79% |

| Early initiation of breastfeeding (within 1 hour of birth) | 56% |
| Infants not weighed at birth | 58% |

International Code of Marketing of Breastmilk Substitutes	Partial
Maternity protection in accordance with ILO Convention 183	No
Exclusive breastfeeding (<6 months)	53%

Timely introduction of complementary foods (with continued breastfeeding)	66%
Continued breastfeeding at two years	35%
Full coverage of vitamin A supplementation	68%
National guidelines for management of severe acute malnutrition incorporating the community-based approach	NA*
Policy on new ORS formula and zinc for management of diarrhoea	Yes
Policy on community treatment of pneumonia with antibiotics	No

To increase children's chances of survival, improve development and prevent stunting, nutrition interventions need to be delivered during the mother's pregnancy and the first two years of the child's life.

*NA: Not applicable

MATERNAL NUTRITION/HEALTH

Maternal mortality ratio, adjusted (per 100,000 live births)	130	(2005)
Maternal mortality ratio, reported (per 100,000 live births)	84	(2000)
Total number of maternal deaths	2,400	(2005)
Lifetime risk of maternal death (1 in :)	230	(2005)
Women with low BMI (<18.5 kg/m², %)	2	(2008)
Anaemia, non-pregnant women (<120 g/l, %)	41	(2005)
Antenatal care (at least one visit, %)	74	(2008)
Antenatal care (at least four visits, %)	66	(2008)
Skilled attendant at birth (%)	79	(2008)
Low birthweight (<2,500 grams, %)	13	(2008)
Primary school net enrolment or attendance ratio (% female, % male)	94, 98	(2007)
Gender parity index (primary school net enrolment or attendance ratio)	0.96	(2007)

WATER AND SANITATION

Drinking water coverage
Percentage of population by type of drinking water source, 2006

Legend: Piped into dwelling, plot or yard; Other improved source; Unimproved source

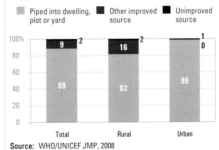

Source: WHO/UNICEF JMP, 2008

Sanitation coverage
Percentage of population by type of sanitation facility, 2006

Legend: Improved facility; Shared facility; Unimproved facility; Open defecation

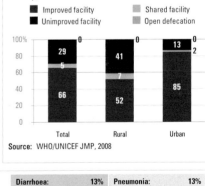

Source: WHO/UNICEF JMP, 2008

Under-five deaths (post-neonatal) caused by: Diarrhoea: 13% Pneumonia: 13%

DISPARITIES IN NUTRITION

Indicator	Gender			Residence			Wealth quintile						Source
	Male	Female	Ratio of male to female	Urban	Rural	Ratio of urban to rural	Poorest	Second	Middle	Fourth	Richest	Ratio of richest to poorest	
Stunting prevalence (WHO Child Growth Standards, %)	31	27	1.1	27	30	0.9	30	31	27	30	27	0.9	DHS 2008
Underweight prevalence (WHO Child Growth Standards, %)	7	5	1.4	6	6	1.0	8	6	6	5	5	0.6	DHS 2008
Wasting prevalence (WHO Child Growth Standards, %)	8	6	1.3	8	7	1.1	7	8	8	6	8	1.1	DHS 2008
Infants not weighed at birth (%)	-	-	-	44	68	0.6	74	71	61	50	33	0.4	DHS 2008
Early initiation of breastfeeding (%)	55	57	1.0	51	59	0.9	60	59	57	56	47	0.8	DHS 2008
Women with low BMI (<18.5 kg/m², %)	-	2	-	1	2	0.5	3	1	1	1	1	0.3	DHS 2008

ETHIOPIA

DEMOGRAPHICS

Total population (000)	80,713	(2008)
Total under-five population (000)	13,323	(2008)
Total number of births (000)	3,093	(2008)
Under-five mortality rate (per 1,000 live births)	109	(2008)
Total number of under-five deaths (000)	321	(2008)
Infant mortality rate (per 1,000 live births)	69	(2008)
Neonatal mortality rate (per 1,000 live births)	41	(2004)
HIV prevalence rate (15–49 years, %)	2.1	(2007)
Population below international poverty line of US$1.25 per day (%)	39	(2005)

Under-five mortality rate
Deaths per 1,000 live births

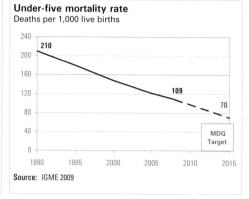

Source: IGME 2009

Causes of under-five deaths, 2004

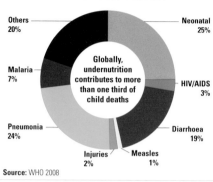

Globally, undernutrition contributes to more than one third of child deaths

- Others 20%
- Neonatal 25%
- Malaria 7%
- HIV/AIDS 3%
- Pneumonia 24%
- Diarrhoea 19%
- Injuries 2%
- Measles 1%

Source: WHO 2008

NUTRITIONAL STATUS

Burden of undernutrition (2008)
WHO Child Growth Standards

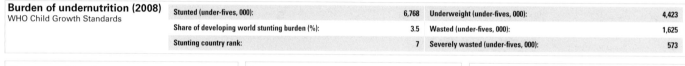

Stunted (under-fives, 000):	6,768	Underweight (under-fives, 000):	4,423
Share of developing world stunting burden (%):	3.5	Wasted (under-fives, 000):	1,625
Stunting country rank:	7	Severely wasted (under-fives, 000):	573

Current nutritional status
Percentage of children < 5 years old suffering from:

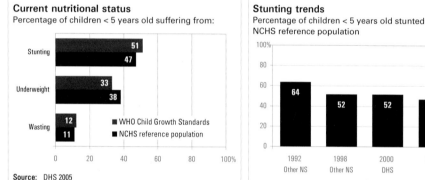

- Stunting: 51 / 47
- Underweight: 33 / 38
- Wasting: 12 / 11

■ WHO Child Growth Standards
■ NCHS reference population

Source: DHS 2005

Stunting trends
Percentage of children < 5 years old stunted NCHS reference population

- 1992 Other NS: 64
- 1998 Other NS: 52
- 2000 DHS: 52
- 2005 DHS: 47

Underweight trends
Percentage of children < 5 years old underweight NCHS reference population

Insufficient progress towards MDG1

- 1992 Other NS: 48
- 1998 Other NS: 44
- 2000 DHS: 47
- 2005 DHS: 38

INFANT AND YOUNG CHILD FEEDING

Infant feeding practices, by age

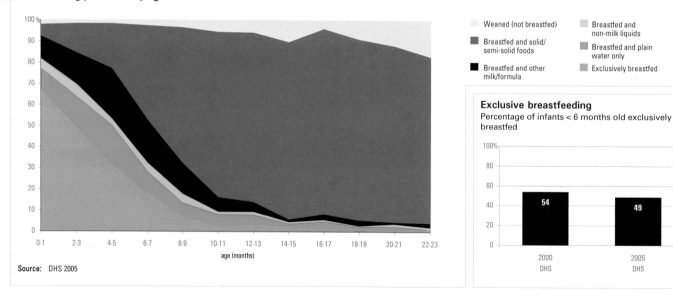

Legend:
- Weaned (not breastfed)
- Breastfed and non-milk liquids
- Breastfed and solid/semi-solid foods
- Breastfed and plain water only
- Breastfed and other milk/formula
- Exclusively breastfed

age (months)

Source: DHS 2005

Exclusive breastfeeding
Percentage of infants < 6 months old exclusively breastfed

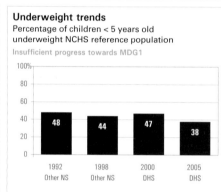

- 2000 DHS: 54
- 2005 DHS: 49

MICRONUTRIENTS

Vitamin A supplementation
Percentage of children 6-59 months old receiving two doses of vitamin A during calendar year

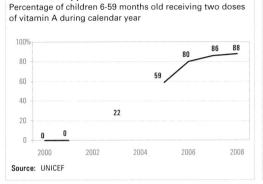

Source: UNICEF

Iodized salt consumption trends*
Percentage of households consuming adequately iodized salt
2,478,000 newborns are unprotected against IDD (2008)

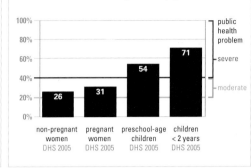

	1995 MICS	2000 DHS	2005 DHS
	0	28	20

* Estimates may not be comparable.

Anaemia
Prevalence of anaemia among selected population

non-pregnant women DHS 2005	pregnant women DHS 2005	preschool-age children DHS 2005	children < 2 years DHS 2005
26	31	54	71

public health problem — severe / moderate

ESSENTIAL NUTRITION INTERVENTIONS DURING THE LIFE CYCLE

| Pregnancy > | Birth > | 0-5 months > | 6-23 months > | 24-59 months > |

Use of iron-folic acid supplements	0%	Early initiation of breastfeeding (within 1 hour of birth)	69%
Household consumption of adequately iodized salt	20%	Infants not weighed at birth	97%

International Code of Marketing of Breastmilk Substitutes	Partial
Maternity protection in accordance with ILO Convention 183	No
Exclusive breastfeeding (<6 months)	49%

Timely introduction of complementary foods (with continued breastfeeding)	54%
Continued breastfeeding at two years	88%

Full coverage of vitamin A supplementation	88%
National guidelines for management of severe acute malnutrition incorporating the community-based approach	Yes
Policy on new ORS formula and zinc for management of diarrhoea	Yes
Policy on community treatment of pneumonia with antibiotics	No

To increase children's chances of survival, improve development and prevent stunting, nutrition interventions need to be delivered during the mother's pregnancy and the first two years of the child's life.

MATERNAL NUTRITION/HEALTH

Maternal mortality ratio, adjusted (per 100,000 live births)	720	(2005)
Maternal mortality ratio, reported (per 100,000 live births)	670	(1998-2004)
Total number of maternal deaths	22,000	(2005)
Lifetime risk of maternal death (1 in :)	27	(2005)
Women with low BMI (<18.5 kg/m², %)	27	(2005)
Anaemia, non-pregnant women (<120 g/l, %)	26	(2005)
Antenatal care (at least one visit, %)	28	(2005)
Antenatal care (at least four visits, %)	12	(2005)
Skilled attendant at birth (%)	6	(2005)
Low birthweight (<2,500 grams, %)	20	(2005)
Primary school net enrolment or attendance ratio (% female, % male)	45, 45	(2005)
Gender parity index (primary school net enrolment or attendance ratio)	1.00	(2005)

WATER AND SANITATION

Drinking water coverage
Percentage of population by type of drinking water source, 2006

Piped into dwelling, plot or yard / Other improved source / Unimproved source

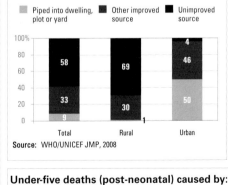

	Total	Rural	Urban
Unimproved source	58	69	4
Other improved source	33	30	46
Piped into dwelling, plot or yard	9	1	50

Source: WHO/UNICEF JMP, 2008

Sanitation coverage
Percentage of population by type of sanitation facility, 2006

Improved facility / Shared facility / Unimproved facility / Open defecation

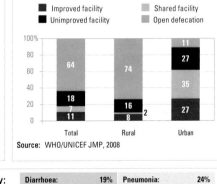

	Total	Rural	Urban
Open defecation	64	74	11
Unimproved facility	18	16	27
Shared facility	7	2	35
Improved facility	11	8	27

Source: WHO/UNICEF JMP, 2008

Under-five deaths (post-neonatal) caused by: Diarrhoea: 19% Pneumonia: 24%

DISPARITIES IN NUTRITION

Indicator	Gender			Residence			Wealth quintile						Source
	Male	Female	Ratio of male to female	Urban	Rural	Ratio of urban to rural	Poorest	Second	Middle	Fourth	Richest	Ratio of richest to poorest	
Stunting prevalence (WHO Child Growth Standards, %)	52	49	1.1	36	52	0.7	53	55	52	51	40	0.8	DHS 2005
Underweight prevalence (WHO Child Growth Standards, %)	34	32	1.1	17	35	0.5	36	39	33	30	25	0.7	DHS 2005
Wasting prevalence (WHO Child Growth Standards, %)	13	11	1.2	8	13	0.6	14	16	12	9	8	0.6	DHS 2005
Infants not weighed at birth (%)	-	-	-	-	-	-	-	-	-	-	-	-	-
Early initiation of breastfeeding (%)	68	70	1.0	65	70	0.9	72	70	70	67	66	0.9	DHS 2005
Women with low BMI (<18.5 kg/m², %)	-	27	-	19	28	0.7	30	30	29	27	20	0.7	DHS 2005

INDIA

DEMOGRAPHICS

Total population (000)	1,181,412	(2008)
Total under-five population (000)	126,642	(2008)
Total number of births (000)	26,913	(2008)
Under-five mortality rate (per 1,000 live births)	69	(2008)
Total number of under-five deaths (000)	1,830	(2008)
Infant mortality rate (per 1,000 live births)	52	(2008)
Neonatal mortality rate (per 1,000 live births)	39	(2004)
HIV prevalence rate (15–49 years, %)	0.3	(2007)
Population below international poverty line of US$1.25 per day (%)	42	(2004-2005)

Under-five mortality rate
Deaths per 1,000 live births

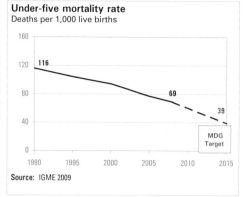

Source: IGME 2009

Causes of under-five deaths, 2004

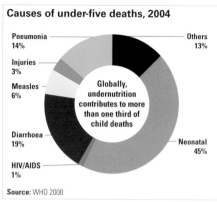

Pneumonia 14%
Injuries 3%
Measles 6%
Diarrhoea 19%
HIV/AIDS 1%
Others 13%
Neonatal 45%

Globally, undernutrition contributes to more than one third of child deaths

Source: WHO 2008

NUTRITIONAL STATUS

Burden of undernutrition (2008)
WHO Child Growth Standards

Stunted (under-fives, 000):	60,788		Underweight (under-fives, 000):	53,823
Share of developing world stunting burden (%):	31.2		Wasted (under-fives, 000):	25,075
Stunting country rank:	1		Severely wasted (under-fives, 000):	8,105

Current nutritional status
Percentage of children < 5 years old suffering from:

Stunting 48 / 43
Underweight 43 / 48
Wasting 20 / 17

■ WHO Child Growth Standards
■ NCHS reference population

Source: NFHS 2005-2006

Stunting trends
Percentage of children < 5 years old stunted NCHS reference population

1992-1993 NFHS: 52
1998-1999 NFHS: 50
2005-2006 NFHS: 43

Underweight trends
Percentage of children < 5 years old underweight NCHS reference population

Insufficient progress towards MDG1

1992-1993 NFHS: 54
1998-1999 NFHS: 49
2005-2006 NFHS: 48

INFANT AND YOUNG CHILD FEEDING

Infant feeding practices, by age

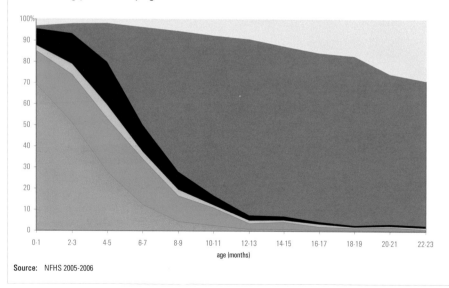

Weaned (not breastfed)
Breastfed and solid/ semi-solid foods
Breastfed and other milk/formula
Breastfed and non-milk liquids
Breastfed and plain water only
Exclusively breastfed

age (months)

Source: NFHS 2005-2006

Exclusive breastfeeding
Percentage of infants < 6 months old exclusively breastfed

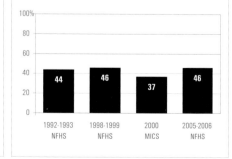

1992-1993 NFHS: 44
1998-1999 NFHS: 46
2000 MICS: 37
2005-2006 NFHS: 46

MICRONUTRIENTS

Vitamin A supplementation
Percentage of children 6-59 months old receiving two doses of vitamin A during calendar year

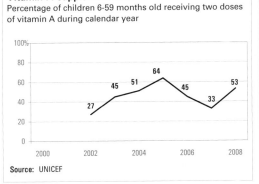

Source: UNICEF

Iodized salt consumption trends*
Percentage of households consuming adequately iodized salt
13,160,000 newborns are unprotected against IDD (2008)

1998-1999 NFHS	49
2000 MICS	50
2005-2006 NFHS	51

* Estimates may not be comparable.

Anaemia
Prevalence of anaemia among selected population

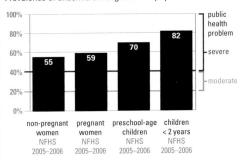

Population	Prevalence
non-pregnant women NFHS 2005–2006	55
pregnant women NFHS 2005–2006	59
preschool-age children NFHS 2005–2006	70
children < 2 years NFHS 2005–2006	82

public health problem / severe / moderate

ESSENTIAL NUTRITION INTERVENTIONS DURING THE LIFE CYCLE

Pregnancy	Birth	0-5 months	6-23 months	24-59 months

Use of iron-folic acid supplements	23%	
Early initiation of breastfeeding (within 1 hour of birth)		25%

International Code of Marketing of Breastmilk Substitutes	Yes
Maternity protection in accordance with ILO Convention 183	No

Household consumption of adequately iodized salt	51%	
Infants not weighed at birth		66%
Exclusive breastfeeding (<6 months)	46%	

Timely introduction of complementary foods (with continued breastfeeding)	57%
Continued breastfeeding at two years	77%
Full coverage of vitamin A supplementation	53%
National guidelines for management of severe acute malnutrition incorporating the community-based approach	No
Policy on new ORS formula and zinc for management of diarrhoea	Yes
Policy on community treatment of pneumonia with antibiotics	Yes

To increase children's chances of survival, improve development and prevent stunting, nutrition interventions need to be delivered during the mother's pregnancy and the first two years of the child's life.

MATERNAL NUTRITION/HEALTH

Maternal mortality ratio, adjusted (per 100,000 live births)	450	(2005)
Maternal mortality ratio, reported (per 100,000 live births)	250	(2001-2003)
Total number of maternal deaths	117,000	(2005)
Lifetime risk of maternal death (1 in :)	70	(2005)
Women with low BMI (<18.5 kg/m², %)	36	(2005-2006)
Anaemia, non-pregnant women (<120 g/l, %)	55	(2005-2006)
Antenatal care (at least one visit, %)	74	(2005-2006)
Antenatal care (at least four visits, %)	37	(2005-2006)
Skilled attendant at birth (%)	47	(2005-2006)
Low birthweight (<2,500 grams, %)	28	(2005-2006)
Primary school net enrolment or attendance ratio (% female, % male)	81, 85	(2005-2006)
Gender parity index (primary school net enrolment or attendance ratio)	0.95	(2005-2006)

WATER AND SANITATION

Drinking water coverage
Percentage of population by type of drinking water source, 2006

Piped into dwelling, plot or yard · Other improved source · Unimproved source

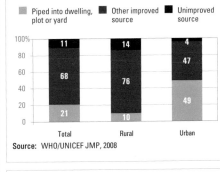

	Total	Rural	Urban
Unimproved source	11	14	4
Other improved source	68	76	47
Piped into dwelling, plot or yard	21	10	49

Source: WHO/UNICEF JMP, 2008

Sanitation coverage
Percentage of population by type of sanitation facility, 2006

Improved facility · Shared facility · Unimproved facility · Open defecation

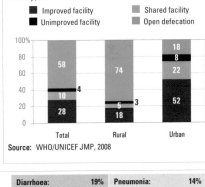

	Total	Rural	Urban
Open defecation	58	74	18
Shared facility			8
Unimproved facility	4	3	22
Improved facility	10 / 28	5 / 18	52

Source: WHO/UNICEF JMP, 2008

Under-five deaths (post-neonatal) caused by:	Diarrhoea:	19%	Pneumonia:	14%

DISPARITIES IN NUTRITION

Indicator	Gender			Residence			Wealth quintile						Source
	Male	Female	Ratio of male to female	Urban	Rural	Ratio of urban to rural	Poorest	Second	Middle	Fourth	Richest	Ratio of richest to poorest	
Stunting prevalence (WHO Child Growth Standards, %)	48	48	1.0	40	51	0.8	60	54	49	41	25	0.4	NFHS 2005-2006
Underweight prevalence (WHO Child Growth Standards, %)	42	43	1.0	33	46	0.7	57	49	41	34	20	0.4	NFHS 2005-2006
Wasting prevalence (WHO Child Growth Standards, %)	21	19	1.1	17	21	0.8	25	22	19	17	13	0.5	NFHS 2005-2006
Infants not weighed at birth (%)	-	-	-	40	75	0.5	89	80	66	49	24	0.3	NFHS 2005-2006
Early initiation of breastfeeding (%)	25	24	1.0	30	22	1.4	17	20	26	28	31	1.8	NFHS 2005-2006
Women with low BMI (<18.5 kg/m², %)	-	36	-	25	41	0.6	52	46	38	29	18	0.3	NFHS 2005-2006

DEMOGRAPHICS

Total population (000)	227,345	(2008)
Total under-five population (000)	20,891	(2008)
Total number of births (000)	4,220	(2008)
Under-five mortality rate (per 1,000 live births)	41	(2008)
Total number of under-five deaths (000)	173	(2008)
Infant mortality rate (per 1,000 live births)	31	(2008)
Neonatal mortality rate (per 1,000 live births)	17	(2004)
HIV prevalence rate (15–49 years, %)	0.2	(2007)
Population below international poverty line of US$1.25 per day (%)	-	-

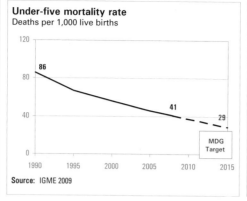

Under-five mortality rate
Deaths per 1,000 live births

Source: IGME 2009

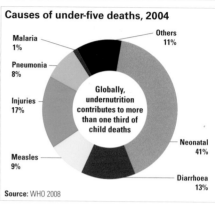

Causes of under-five deaths, 2004

Globally, undernutrition contributes to more than one third of child deaths

- Malaria 1%
- Pneumonia 8%
- Injuries 17%
- Measles 9%
- Others 11%
- Neonatal 41%
- Diarrhoea 13%

Source: WHO 2008

NUTRITIONAL STATUS

Burden of undernutrition (2008)
WHO Child Growth Standards

Stunted (under-fives, 000):	7,688	Underweight (under-fives, 000):	3,844
Share of developing world stunting burden (%):	3.9	Wasted (under-fives, 000):	2,841
Stunting country rank:	5	Severely wasted (under-fives, 000):	1,295

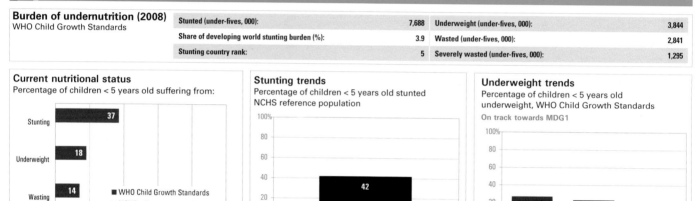

Current nutritional status
Percentage of children < 5 years old suffering from:

- Stunting 37
- Underweight 18
- Wasting 14

■ WHO Child Growth Standards
■ NCHS reference population

Source: Other NS 2007

Stunting trends
Percentage of children < 5 years old stunted
NCHS reference population

- 1995 MICS: 42

Underweight trends
Percentage of children < 5 years old underweight, WHO Child Growth Standards
On track towards MDG1

- 1995 Other NS: 27
- 2003 Other NS: 23
- 2007 Other NS: 18

INFANT AND YOUNG CHILD FEEDING

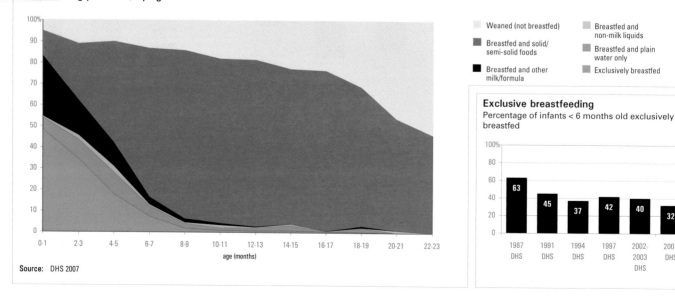

Infant feeding practices, by age

- Weaned (not breastfed)
- Breastfed and solid/semi-solid foods
- Breastfed and other milk/formula
- Breastfed and non-milk liquids
- Breastfed and plain water only
- Exclusively breastfed

age (months)

Source: DHS 2007

Exclusive breastfeeding
Percentage of infants < 6 months old exclusively breastfed

- 1987 DHS: 63
- 1991 DHS: 45
- 1994 DHS: 37
- 1997 DHS: 42
- 2002-2003 DHS: 40
- 2007 DHS: 32

MICRONUTRIENTS

Vitamin A supplementation
Percentage of children 6-59 months old receiving two doses of vitamin A during calendar year

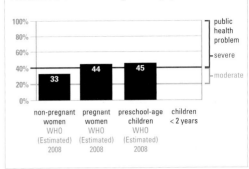

Values: 68 (2000), 57, 63, 62, 73, 76, 82, 87, 86 (2008)

Source: UNICEF

Iodized salt consumption trends*
Percentage of households consuming adequately iodized salt
1,591,000 newborns are unprotected against IDD (2008)

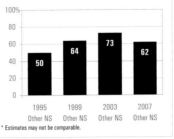

1995	1999	2003	2007
50	64	73	62
Other NS	Other NS	Other NS	Other NS

* Estimates may not be comparable.

Anaemia
Prevalence of anaemia among selected population

non-pregnant women WHO (Estimated) 2008	pregnant women WHO (Estimated) 2008	preschool-age children WHO (Estimated) 2008	children < 2 years
33	44	45	

public health problem — severe — moderate

ESSENTIAL NUTRITION INTERVENTIONS DURING THE LIFE CYCLE

Pregnancy	Birth	0-5 months	6-23 months	24-59 months

Use of iron-folic acid supplements	29%	Early initiation of breastfeeding (within 1 hour of birth)	39%	International Code of Marketing of Breastmilk Substitutes	Partial

				Maternity protection in accordance with ILO Convention 183	No

Household consumption of adequately iodized salt	62%	Infants not weighed at birth	17%	Exclusive breastfeeding (<6 months)	32%	Timely introduction of complementary foods (with continued breastfeeding)	75%

Continued breastfeeding at two years — 50%

Full coverage of vitamin A supplementation — 86%

National guidelines for management of severe acute malnutrition incorporating the community-based approach — No

Policy on new ORS formula and zinc for management of diarrhoea — Yes

Policy on community treatment of pneumonia with antibiotics — No

To increase children's chances of survival, improve development and prevent stunting, nutrition interventions need to be delivered during the mother's pregnancy and the first two years of the child's life.

MATERNAL NUTRITION/HEALTH

Maternal mortality ratio, adjusted (per 100,000 live births)	420	(2005)
Maternal mortality ratio, reported (per 100,000 live births)	230	(2007)
Total number of maternal deaths	19,000	(2005)
Lifetime risk of maternal death (1 in :)	97	(2005)
Women with low BMI (<18.5 kg/m², %)	-	-
Anaemia, non-pregnant women (<120 g/l, %)	33	(2008)
Antenatal care (at least one visit, %)	93	(2007)
Antenatal care (at least four visits, %)	82	(2007)
Skilled attendant at birth (%)	79	(2007)
Low birthweight (<2,500 grams, %)	9	(2007)
Primary school net enrolment or attendance ratio (% female, % male)	84, 86	(2007)
Gender parity index (primary school net enrolment or attendance ratio)	0.98	(2007)

WATER AND SANITATION

Drinking water coverage
Percentage of population by type of drinking water source, 2006

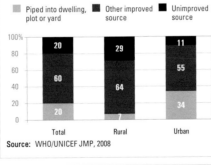

Legend: Piped into dwelling, plot or yard; Other improved source; Unimproved source

	Total	Rural	Urban
Unimproved source	20	29	11
Other improved source	60	64	55
Piped into dwelling, plot or yard	20	7	34

Source: WHO/UNICEF JMP, 2008

Sanitation coverage
Percentage of population by type of sanitation facility, 2006

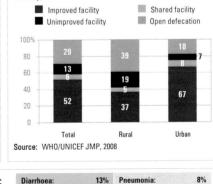

Legend: Improved facility; Shared facility; Unimproved facility; Open defecation

	Total	Rural	Urban
Open defecation	29	39	18
Shared facility	13	19	7/8
Unimproved facility	6	5	
Improved facility	52	37	67

Source: WHO/UNICEF JMP, 2008

Under-five deaths (post-neonatal) caused by: Diarrhoea: 13% Pneumonia: 8%

DISPARITIES IN NUTRITION

Indicator	Gender			Residence			Wealth quintile						Source
	Male	Female	Ratio of male to female	Urban	Rural	Ratio of urban to rural	Poorest	Second	Middle	Fourth	Richest	Ratio of richest to poorest	
Stunting prevalence (WHO Child Growth Standards, %)	-	-	-	-	-	-	-	-	-	-	-	-	
Underweight prevalence (WHO Child Growth Standards, %)	26	21	1.2	21	25	0.8	-	-	-	-	-	-	Other NS 2003
Wasting prevalence (WHO Child Growth Standards, %)	-	-	-	-	-	-	-	-	-	-	-	-	
Infants not weighed at birth (%)	-	-	-	5	27	0.2	44	20	9	4	1	0.0	DHS 2007
Early initiation of breastfeeding (%)	38	40	1.0	39	40	1.0	48	42	38	35	25	0.5	Other NS 2007
Women with low BMI (<18.5 kg/m², %)	-	-	-	-	-	-	-	-	-	-	-	-	

KENYA

DEMOGRAPHICS

Total population (000)	38,765	(2008)
Total under-five population (000)	6,540	(2008)
Total number of births (000)	1,506	(2008)
Under-five mortality rate (per 1,000 live births)	128	(2008)
Total number of under-five deaths (000)	189	(2008)
Infant mortality rate (per 1,000 live births)	81	(2008)
Neonatal mortality rate (per 1,000 live births)	34	(2004)
HIV prevalence rate (15–49 years, %)	-	
Population below international poverty line of US$1.25 per day (%)	20	(2005-2006)

Under-five mortality rate
Deaths per 1,000 live births

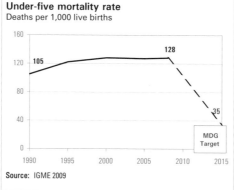

Source: IGME 2009

Causes of under-five deaths, 2004

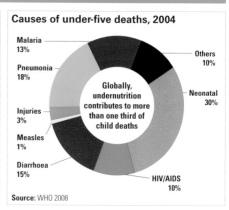

Malaria 13%
Pneumonia 18%
Injuries 3%
Measles 1%
Diarrhoea 15%
Others 10%
Neonatal 30%
HIV/AIDS 10%

Globally, undernutrition contributes to more than one third of child deaths

Source: WHO 2008

NUTRITIONAL STATUS

Burden of undernutrition (2008)
NCHS reference population

Stunted (under-fives, 000):	2,269	Underweight (under-fives, 000):	1,367
Share of developing world stunting burden (%):	1.2	Wasted (under-fives, 000):	412
Stunting country rank:	16	Severely wasted (under-fives, 000):	78

Current nutritional status
Percentage of children < 5 years old suffering from:

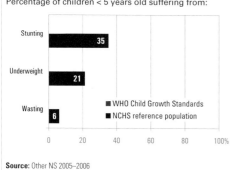

Stunting 35
Underweight 21
Wasting 6

■ WHO Child Growth Standards
■ NCHS reference population

Source: Other NS 2005–2006

Stunting trends
Percentage of children < 5 years old stunted
NCHS reference population

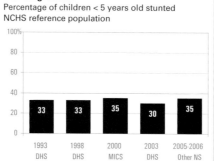

1993 DHS	1998 DHS	2000 MICS	2003 DHS	2005-2006 Other NS
33	33	35	30	35

Underweight trends
Percentage of children < 5 years old underweight NCHS reference population

Insufficient progress towards MDG1

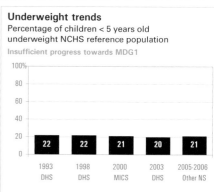

1993 DHS	1998 DHS	2000 MICS	2003 DHS	2005-2006 Other NS
22	22	21	20	21

INFANT AND YOUNG CHILD FEEDING

Infant feeding practices, by age

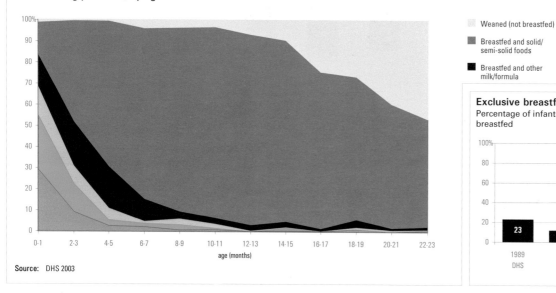

age (months)

■ Weaned (not breastfed)
■ Breastfed and solid/semi-solid foods
■ Breastfed and other milk/formula
■ Breastfed and non-milk liquids
■ Breastfed and plain water only
■ Exclusively breastfed

Source: DHS 2003

Exclusive breastfeeding
Percentage of infants < 6 months old exclusively breastfed

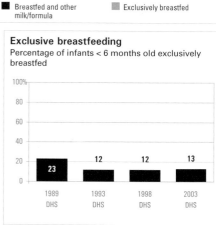

1989 DHS	1993 DHS	1998 DHS	2003 DHS
23	12	12	13

MICRONUTRIENTS

Vitamin A supplementation
Percentage of children 6-59 months old receiving two doses of vitamin A during calendar year

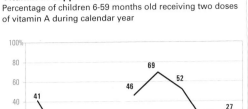

Source: UNICEF

Iodized salt consumption trends*
Percentage of households consuming adequately iodized salt
142,000 newborns are unprotected against IDD (2008)

100	91
1995 Other NS	2000 MICS

* Estimates may not be comparable.

Anaemia
Prevalence of anaemia among selected population

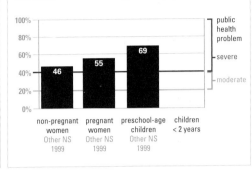

ESSENTIAL NUTRITION INTERVENTIONS DURING THE LIFE CYCLE

Pregnancy	Birth	0-5 months	6-23 months	24-59 months

Use of iron-folic acid supplements	3%	Early initiation of breastfeeding (within 1 hour of birth)	52%

International Code of Marketing of Breastmilk Substitutes	Partial
Maternity protection in accordance with ILO Convention 183	No

Household consumption of adequately iodized salt	91%	Infants not weighed at birth	55%

Exclusive breastfeeding (<6 months)	13%

Timely introduction of complementary foods (with continued breastfeeding)	84%
Continued breastfeeding at two years	57%

Full coverage of vitamin A supplementation	27%
National guidelines for management of severe acute malnutrition incorporating the community-based approach	Yes
Policy on new ORS formula and zinc for management of diarrhoea	Partial
Policy on community treatment of pneumonia with antibiotics	No

To increase children's chances of survival, improve development and prevent stunting, nutrition interventions need to be delivered during the mother's pregnancy and the first two years of the child's life.

MATERNAL NUTRITION/HEALTH

Maternal mortality ratio, adjusted (per 100,000 live births)	560	(2005)
Maternal mortality ratio, reported (per 100,000 live births)	410	(1993-2003)
Total number of maternal deaths	7,700	(2005)
Lifetime risk of maternal death (1 in :)	39	(2005)
Women with low BMI (<18.5 kg/m², %)	12	(2003)
Anaemia, non-pregnant women (<120 g/l, %)	46	(1999)
Antenatal care (at least one visit, %)	88	(2003)
Antenatal care (at least four visits, %)	52	(2003)
Skilled attendant at birth (%)	42	(2003)
Low birthweight (<2,500 grams, %)	10	(2003)
Primary school net enrolment or attendance ratio (% female, % male)	76, 75	(2006)
Gender parity index (primary school net enrolment or attendance ratio)	1.01	(2006)

WATER AND SANITATION

Drinking water coverage
Percentage of population by type of drinking water source, 2006

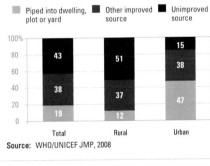

- Piped into dwelling, plot or yard
- Other improved source
- Unimproved source

Source: WHO/UNICEF JMP, 2008

Sanitation coverage
Percentage of population by type of sanitation facility, 2006

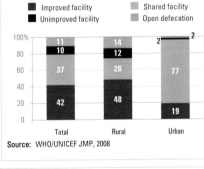

- Improved facility
- Unimproved facility
- Shared facility
- Open defecation

Source: WHO/UNICEF JMP, 2008

Under-five deaths (post-neonatal) caused by:	Diarrhoea:	15%	Pneumonia:	18%

DISPARITIES IN NUTRITION

Indicator	Gender			Residence			Wealth quintile						Source
	Male	Female	Ratio of male to female	Urban	Rural	Ratio of urban to rural	Poorest	Second	Middle	Fourth	Richest	Ratio of richest to poorest	
Stunting prevalence (WHO Child Growth Standards, %)	40	32	1.3	30	37	0.8	45	38	35	33	25	0.6	DHS 2003
Underweight prevalence (WHO Child Growth Standards, %)	19	13	1.5	10	17	0.6	24	16	14	13	7	0.3	DHS 2003
Wasting prevalence (WHO Child Growth Standards, %)	7	5	1.4	5	6	0.8	9	7	4	5	4	0.4	DHS 2003
Infants not weighed at birth (%)	-	-	-	24	62	0.4	79	65	56	41	21	0.3	DHS 2003
Early initiation of breastfeeding (%)	51	54	0.9	51	53	1.0	50	54	52	55	52	1.0	DHS 2003
Women with low BMI (<18.5 kg/m², %)	-	12	-	5	15	0.3	23	17	12	10	5	0.2	DHS 2003

MADAGASCAR

DEMOGRAPHICS

Total population (000)	19,111	(2008)
Total under-five population (000)	3,060	(2008)
Total number of births (000)	687	(2008)
Under-five mortality rate (per 1,000 live births)	106	(2008)
Total number of under-five deaths (000)	71	(2008)
Infant mortality rate (per 1,000 live births)	68	(2008)
Neonatal mortality rate (per 1,000 live births)	41	(2004)
HIV prevalence rate (15–49 years, %)	0.1	(2007)
Population below international poverty line of US$1.25 per day (%)	68	(2005)

Under-five mortality rate
Deaths per 1,000 live births

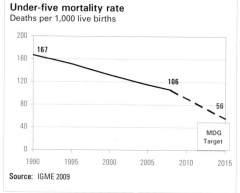

Source: IGME 2009

Causes of under-five deaths, 2004

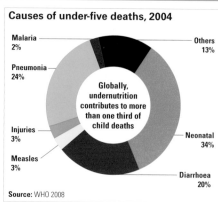

Malaria 2%
Pneumonia 24%
Injuries 3%
Measles 3%
Others 13%
Neonatal 34%
Diarrhoea 20%

Globally, undernutrition contributes to more than one third of child deaths

Source: WHO 2008

NUTRITIONAL STATUS

Burden of undernutrition (2008)
WHO Child Growth Standards

Stunted (under-fives, 000):	1,622	Underweight (under-fives, 000):	1,093
Share of developing world stunting burden (%):	0.8	Wasted (under-fives, 000):	459
Stunting country rank:	21	Severely wasted (under-fives, 000):	162

Current nutritional status
Percentage of children < 5 years old suffering from:

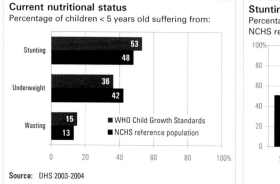

Stunting: 53 / 48
Underweight: 36 / 42
Wasting: 15 / 13

■ WHO Child Growth Standards
■ NCHS reference population

Source: DHS 2003-2004

Stunting trends
Percentage of children < 5 years old stunted
NCHS reference population

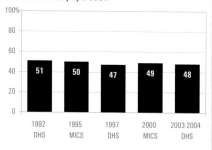

1992 DHS	1995 MICS	1997 DHS	2000 MICS	2003-2004 DHS
51	50	47	49	48

Underweight trends
Percentage of children < 5 years old
underweight NCHS reference population

No progress towards MDG1

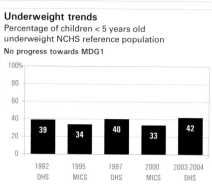

1992 DHS	1995 MICS	1997 DHS	2000 MICS	2003-2004 DHS
39	34	40	33	42

INFANT AND YOUNG CHILD FEEDING

Infant feeding practices, by age

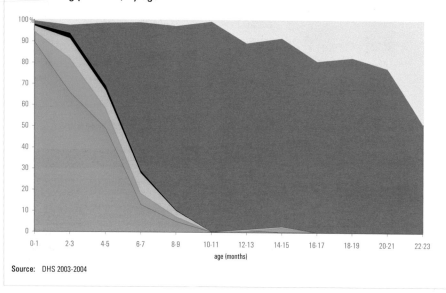

□ Weaned (not breastfed)
■ Breastfed and solid/semi-solid foods
■ Breastfed and other milk/formula
□ Breastfed and non-milk liquids
■ Breastfed and plain water only
■ Exclusively breastfed

Source: DHS 2003-2004

Exclusive breastfeeding
Percentage of infants < 6 months old exclusively breastfed

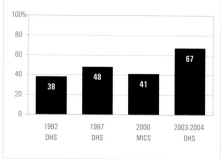

1992 DHS	1997 DHS	2000 MICS	2003-2004 DHS
38	48	41	67

MICRONUTRIENTS

Vitamin A supplementation
Percentage of children 6-59 months old receiving two doses of vitamin A during calendar year

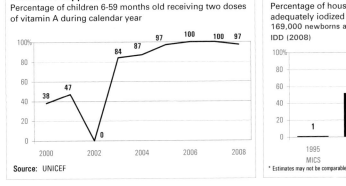

Source: UNICEF

Iodized salt consumption trends*
Percentage of households consuming adequately iodized salt
169,000 newborns are unprotected against IDD (2008)

1	52	75
1995 MICS	2000 MICS	2003-2004 DHS

* Estimates may not be comparable.

Anaemia
Prevalence of anaemia among selected population

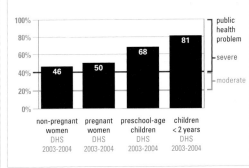

non-pregnant women DHS 2003-2004	pregnant women DHS 2003-2004	preschool-age children DHS 2003-2004	children < 2 years DHS 2003-2004
46	50	68	81

- public health problem
- severe
- moderate

ESSENTIAL NUTRITION INTERVENTIONS DURING THE LIFE CYCLE

| Pregnancy | Birth | 0-5 months | 6-23 months | 24-59 months |

Use of iron-folic acid supplements	3%	Early initiation of breastfeeding (within 1 hour of birth)	62%
Household consumption of adequately iodized salt	75%	Infants not weighed at birth	61%

International Code of Marketing of Breastmilk Substitutes	Partial
Maternity protection in accordance with ILO Convention 183	No
Exclusive breastfeeding (<6 months)	67%

Timely introduction of complementary foods (with continued breastfeeding)	78%
Continued breastfeeding at two years	64%

Full coverage of vitamin A supplementation	97%
National guidelines for management of severe acute malnutrition incorporating the community-based approach	Yes
Policy on new ORS formula and zinc for management of diarrhoea	Yes
Policy on community treatment of pneumonia with antibiotics	Yes

To increase children's chances of survival, improve development and prevent stunting, nutrition interventions need to be delivered during the mother's pregnancy and the first two years of the child's life.

MATERNAL NUTRITION/HEALTH

Maternal mortality ratio, adjusted (per 100,000 live births)	510	(2005)
Maternal mortality ratio, reported (per 100,000 live births)	470	(1999-2003)
Total number of maternal deaths	3,600	(2005)
Lifetime risk of maternal death (1 in :)	38	(2005)
Women with low BMI (<18.5 kg/m², %)	19	(2003-2004)
Anaemia, non-pregnant women (<120 g/l, %)	46	(2003-2004)
Antenatal care (at least one visit, %)	80	(2003-2004)
Antenatal care (at least four visits, %)	40	(2003-2004)
Skilled attendant at birth (%)	51	(2003-2004)
Low birthweight (<2,500 grams, %)	17	(2003-2004)
Primary school net enrolment or attendance ratio (% female, % male)	77, 74	(2003-2004)
Gender parity index (primary school net enrolment or attendance ratio)	1.04	(2003-2004)

WATER AND SANITATION

Drinking water coverage
Percentage of population by type of drinking water source, 2006

- Piped into dwelling, plot or yard
- Other improved source
- Unimproved source

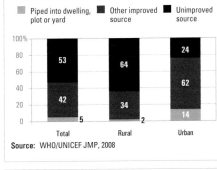

	Total	Rural	Urban
Unimproved	53	64	24
Other improved	42	34	62
Piped	5	2	14

Source: WHO/UNICEF JMP, 2008

Sanitation coverage
Percentage of population by type of sanitation facility, 2006

- Improved facility
- Unimproved facility
- Shared facility
- Open defecation

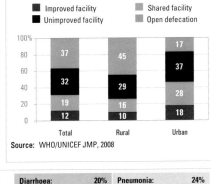

	Total	Rural	Urban
Open defecation	37	45	17
Shared	32	29	37
Unimproved	19	16	28
Improved	12	10	18

Source: WHO/UNICEF JMP, 2008

Under-five deaths (post-neonatal) caused by:	Diarrhoea:	20%	Pneumonia:	24%

DISPARITIES IN NUTRITION

Indicator	Gender			Residence			Wealth quintile						Source
	Male	Female	Ratio of male to female	Urban	Rural	Ratio of urban to rural	Poorest	Second	Middle	Fourth	Richest	Ratio of richest to poorest	
Stunting prevalence (WHO Child Growth Standards, %)	55	51	1.1	46	55	0.8	59	58	53	47	44	0.7	DHS 2003-2004
Underweight prevalence (WHO Child Growth Standards, %)	38	33	1.2	31	37	0.8	40	41	39	29	24	0.6	DHS 2003-2004
Wasting prevalence (WHO Child Growth Standards, %)	18	12	1.5	14	15	0.9	16	15	15	15	13	0.8	DHS 2003-2004
Infants not weighed at birth (%)	-	-	-	42	65	0.6	77	74	64	49	23	0.3	DHS 2003-2004
Early initiation of breastfeeding (%)	61	64	1.0	72	60	1.2	58	60	59	65	77	1.3	DHS 2003-2004
Women with low BMI (<18.5 kg/m², %)	-	19	-	15	21	0.7	28	26	20	18	9	0.3	DHS 2003-2004

MEXICO

Total population (000)	108,555	(2008)
Total under-five population (000)	10,281	(2008)
Total number of births (000)	2,049	(2008)
Under-five mortality rate (per 1,000 live births)	17	(2008)
Total number of under-five deaths (000)	36	(2008)
Infant mortality rate (per 1,000 live births)	15	(2008)
Neonatal mortality rate (per 1,000 live births)	11	(2004)
HIV prevalence rate (15–49 years, %)	0.3	(2007)
Population below international poverty line of US$1.25 per day (%)	<2	(2006)

Under-five mortality rate
Deaths per 1,000 live births

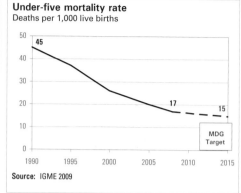

Source: IGME 2009

Causes of under-five deaths, 2004

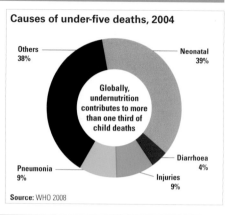

Globally, undernutrition contributes to more than one third of child deaths

Others 38%
Neonatal 39%
Diarrhoea 4%
Injuries 9%
Pneumonia 9%

Source: WHO 2008

NUTRITIONAL STATUS

Burden of undernutrition (2008)
WHO Child Growth Standards

Stunted (under-fives, 000):	1,594	Underweight (under-fives, 000):		350
Share of developing world stunting burden (%):	0.8	Wasted (under-fives, 000):		206
Stunting country rank:	22	Severely wasted (under-fives, 000):		-

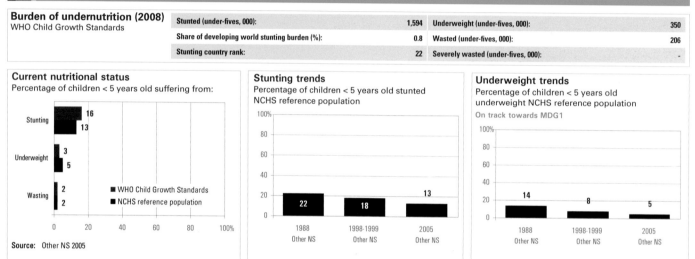

Current nutritional status
Percentage of children < 5 years old suffering from:

Stunting 16 / 13
Underweight 3 / 5
Wasting 2 / 2

■ WHO Child Growth Standards
■ NCHS reference population

Source: Other NS 2005

Stunting trends
Percentage of children < 5 years old stunted
NCHS reference population

1988 Other NS: 22
1998-1999 Other NS: 18
2005 Other NS: 13

Underweight trends
Percentage of children < 5 years old
underweight NCHS reference population
On track towards MDG1

1988 Other NS: 14
1998-1999 Other NS: 8
2005 Other NS: 5

INFANT AND YOUNG CHILD FEEDING

Infant feeding practices, by age

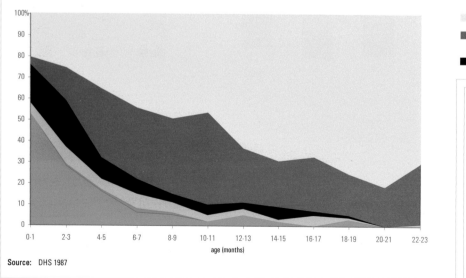

Weaned (not breastfed)
Breastfed and solid/semi-solid foods
Breastfed and other milk/formula
Breastfed and non-milk liquids
Breastfed and plain water only
Exclusively breastfed

Source: DHS 1987

Exclusive breastfeeding
Percentage of infants < 6 months old exclusively breastfed

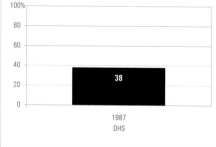

1987 DHS: 38

MICRONUTRIENTS

Vitamin A supplementation
Percentage of children 6-59 months old receiving two doses of vitamin A during calendar year

Subnational Programme

Iodized salt consumption trends*
Percentage of households consuming adequately iodized salt
184,000 newborns are unprotected against IDD (2008)

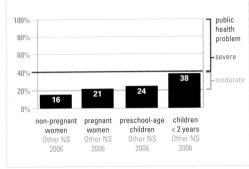

2003
Other NS

* Estimates may not be comparable.

Anaemia
Prevalence of anaemia among selected population

non-pregnant women	16
pregnant women	21
preschool-age children	24
children < 2 years	38

Other NS 2006

public health problem — severe — moderate

ESSENTIAL NUTRITION INTERVENTIONS DURING THE LIFE CYCLE

Pregnancy	Birth	0-5 months	6-23 months	24-59 months

Use of iron-folic acid supplements	-	
Household consumption of adequately iodized salt	91%	

Early initiation of breastfeeding (within 1 hour of birth)	-
Infants not weighed at birth	-

International Code of Marketing of Breastmilk Substitutes	Yes
Maternity protection in accordance with ILO Convention 183	No
Exclusive breastfeeding (<6 months)	38%

Timely introduction of complementary foods (with continued breastfeeding)	36%
Continued breastfeeding at two years	21%
Full coverage of vitamin A supplementation	SP*
National guidelines for management of severe acute malnutrition incorporating the community-based approach	NA*
Policy on new ORS formula and zinc for management of diarrhoea	No
Policy on community treatment of pneumonia with antibiotics	-

To increase children's chances of survival, improve development and prevent stunting, nutrition interventions need to be delivered during the mother's pregnancy and the first two years of the child's life.

*SP: Subnational programme
*NA: Not applicable

MATERNAL NUTRITION/HEALTH

Maternal mortality ratio, adjusted (per 100,000 live births)	60	(2005)
Maternal mortality ratio, reported (per 100,000 live births)	56	(2007)
Total number of maternal deaths	1,300	(2005)
Lifetime risk of maternal death (1 in :)	670	(2005)
Women with low BMI (<18.5 kg/m², %)	-	-
Anaemia, non-pregnant women (<120 g/l, %)	16	(2006)
Antenatal care (at least one visit, %)	94	(2006)
Antenatal care (at least four visits, %)	-	-
Skilled attendant at birth (%)	93	(2006)
Low birthweight (<2,500 grams, %)	8	(2006)
Primary school net enrolment or attendance ratio (% female, % male)	97, 98	(2006)
Gender parity index (primary school net enrolment or attendance ratio)	0.99	(2006)

WATER AND SANITATION

Drinking water coverage
Percentage of population by type of drinking water source, 2006

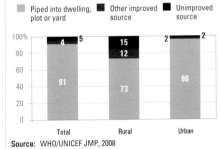

- Piped into dwelling, plot or yard
- Other improved source
- Unimproved source

Source: WHO/UNICEF JMP, 2008

Sanitation coverage
Percentage of population by type of sanitation facility, 2006

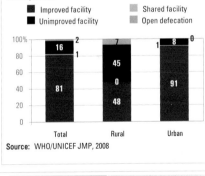

- Improved facility
- Unimproved facility
- Shared facility
- Open defecation

Source: WHO/UNICEF JMP, 2008

Under-five deaths (post-neonatal) caused by:	Diarrhoea:	4%	Pneumonia:	9%

DISPARITIES IN NUTRITION

Indicator	Gender			Residence			Wealth quintile						Source
	Male	Female	Ratio of male to female	Urban	Rural	Ratio of urban to rural	Poorest	Second	Middle	Fourth	Richest	Ratio of richest to poorest	
Stunting prevalence (WHO Child Growth Standards, %)	-	-	-	-	-	-	-	-	-	-	-	-	
Underweight prevalence (NCHS reference population, %)	8	7	1.1	6	12	0.5	-	-	-	-	-	-	Other NS 1998-1999
Wasting prevalence (WHO Child Growth Standards, %)	-	-	-	-	-	-	-	-	-	-	-	-	
Infants not weighed at birth (%)	-	-	-	-	-	-	-	-	-	-	-	-	
Early initiation of breastfeeding (%)	-	-	-	-	-	-	-	-	-	-	-	-	
Women with low BMI (<18.5 kg/m², %)	-	-	-	-	-	-	-	-	-	-	-	-	

MOZAMBIQUE

Total population (000)	22,383	(2008)
Total under-five population (000)	3,820	(2008)
Total number of births (000)	876	(2008)
Under-five mortality rate (per 1,000 live births)	130	(2008)
Total number of under-five deaths (000)	110	(2008)
Infant mortality rate (per 1,000 live births)	90	(2008)
Neonatal mortality rate (per 1,000 live births)	35	(2004)
HIV prevalence rate (15–49 years, %)	12.5	(2007)
Population below international poverty line of US$1.25 per day (%)	75	(2002-2003)

Under-five mortality rate
Deaths per 1,000 live births

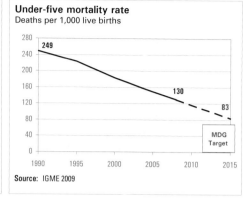

Source: IGME 2009

Causes of under-five deaths, 2004

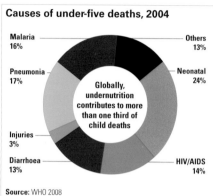

Malaria 16%
Others 13%
Pneumonia 17%
Neonatal 24%
Injuries 3%
Diarrhoea 13%
HIV/AIDS 14%

Globally, undernutrition contributes to more than one third of child deaths

Source: WHO 2008

NUTRITIONAL STATUS

Burden of undernutrition (2008)
NCHS reference population

Stunted (under-fives, 000):	1,670	Underweight (under-fives, 000):	669
Share of developing world stunting burden (%):	0.9	Wasted (under-fives, 000):	160
Stunting country rank:	20	Severely wasted (under-fives, 000):	53

Current nutritional status
Percentage of children < 5 years old suffering from:

Stunting 44
Underweight 18
Wasting 4

■ WHO Child Growth Standards
■ NCHS reference population

Source: MICS 2008

Stunting trends
Percentage of children < 5 years old stunted
NCHS reference population

1995 MICS	1997 DHS	2000 Other NS	2003 DHS	2008 MICS
55	40	44	41	44

Underweight trends
Percentage of children < 5 years old
underweight NCHS reference population
On track towards MDG1

1995 MICS	1997 DHS	2000 Other NS	2003 DHS	2008 MICS
27	24	26	24	18

INFANT AND YOUNG CHILD FEEDING

Infant feeding practices, by age

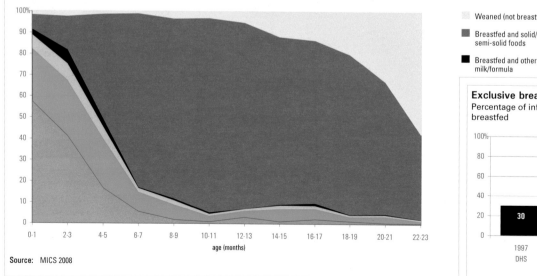

age (months)

Source: MICS 2008

□ Weaned (not breastfed)
■ Breastfed and solid/semi-solid foods
■ Breastfed and other milk/formula
□ Breastfed and non-milk liquids
■ Breastfed and plain water only
■ Exclusively breastfed

Exclusive breastfeeding
Percentage of infants < 6 months old exclusively breastfed

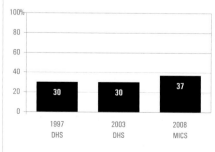

1997 DHS	2003 DHS	2008 MICS
30	30	37

MICRONUTRIENTS

Vitamin A supplementation
Percentage of children 6-59 months old receiving two doses of vitamin A during calendar year

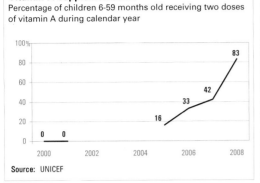

Source: UNICEF

Iodized salt consumption trends*
Percentage of households consuming adequately iodized salt
656,000 newborns are unprotected against IDD (2008)

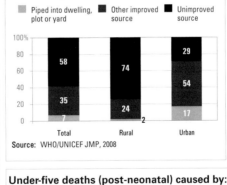

* Estimates may not be comparable.

Anaemia
Prevalence of anaemia among selected population

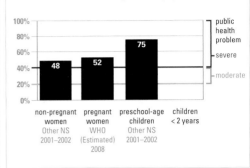

ESSENTIAL NUTRITION INTERVENTIONS DURING THE LIFE CYCLE

Pregnancy	Birth	0-5 months	6-23 months	24-59 months

Use of iron-folic acid supplements	14%	Early initiation of breastfeeding (within 1 hour of birth)	63%

International Code of Marketing of Breastmilk Substitutes	Yes
Maternity protection in accordance with ILO Convention 183	No

Household consumption of adequately iodized salt	25%	Infants not weighed at birth	42%	Exclusive breastfeeding (<6 months)	37%	Timely introduction of complementary foods (with continued breastfeeding)	84%
						Continued breastfeeding at two years	54%

Full coverage of vitamin A supplementation	83%
National guidelines for management of severe acute malnutrition incorporating the community-based approach	Yes
Policy on new ORS formula and zinc for management of diarrhoea	Partial
Policy on community treatment of pneumonia with antibiotics	Partial

To increase children's chances of survival, improve development and prevent stunting, nutrition interventions need to be delivered during the mother's pregnancy and the first two years of the child's life.

MATERNAL NUTRITION/HEALTH

Maternal mortality ratio, adjusted (per 100,000 live births)	520	(2005)
Maternal mortality ratio, reported (per 100,000 live births)	410	(1994-2003)
Total number of maternal deaths	4,000	(2005)
Lifetime risk of maternal death (1 in :)	45	(2005)
Women with low BMI (<18.5 kg/m², %)	9	(2003)
Anaemia, non-pregnant women (<120 g/l, %)	48	(2001-2002)
Antenatal care (at least one visit, %)	89	(2008)
Antenatal care (at least four visits, %)	53	(2003)
Skilled attendant at birth (%)	55	(2008)
Low birthweight (<2,500 grams, %)	15	(2008)
Primary school net enrolment or attendance ratio (% female, % male)	80, 82	(2008)
Gender parity index (primary school net enrolment or attendance ratio)	0.98	(2008)

WATER AND SANITATION

Drinking water coverage
Percentage of population by type of drinking water source, 2006

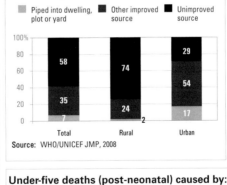

Source: WHO/UNICEF JMP, 2008

Sanitation coverage
Percentage of population by type of sanitation facility, 2006

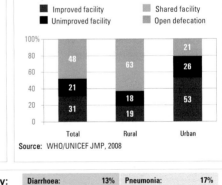

Source: WHO/UNICEF JMP, 2008

Under-five deaths (post-neonatal) caused by:	Diarrhoea:	13%	Pneumonia:	17%

DISPARITIES IN NUTRITION

Indicator	Gender			Residence			Wealth quintile						Source
	Male	Female	Ratio of male to female	Urban	Rural	Ratio of urban to rural	Poorest	Second	Middle	Fourth	Richest	Ratio of richest to poorest	
Stunting prevalence (WHO Child Growth Standards, %)	49	44	1.1	35	52	0.7	54	54	52	41	25	0.5	DHS 2003
Underweight prevalence (WHO Child Growth Standards, %)	21	19	1.1	12	23	0.5	26	24	21	16	7	0.3	DHS 2003
Wasting prevalence (WHO Child Growth Standards, %)	5	5	1.0	4	6	0.7	7	5	4	5	4	0.6	DHS 2003
Infants not weighed at birth (%)	-	-	-	17	52	0.3	61	53	45	30	6	0.1	MICS 2008
Early initiation of breastfeeding (%)	-	-	-	60	64	0.9	68	66	64	55	60	0.9	MICS 2008
Women with low BMI (<18.5 kg/m², %)	-	9	-	6	10	0.6	10	12	10	7	5	0.5	DHS 2003

MYANMAR

DEMOGRAPHICS

Total population (000)	49,563	(2008)
Total under-five population (000)	4,629	(2008)
Total number of births (000)	1,020	(2008)
Under-five mortality rate (per 1,000 live births)	98	(2008)
Total number of under-five deaths (000)	98	(2008)
Infant mortality rate (per 1,000 live births)	71	(2008)
Neonatal mortality rate (per 1,000 live births)	49	(2004)
HIV prevalence rate (15–49 years, %)	0.7	(2007)
Population below international poverty line of US$1.25 per day (%)	-	

Under-five mortality rate
Deaths per 1,000 live births

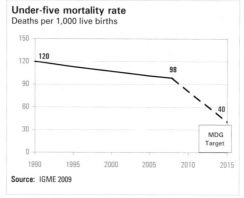

Source: IGME 2009

Causes of under-five deaths, 2004

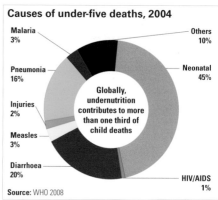

Malaria 3%
Pneumonia 16%
Injuries 2%
Measles 3%
Diarrhoea 20%
Others 10%
Neonatal 45%
HIV/AIDS 1%

Globally, undernutrition contributes to more than one third of child deaths

Source: WHO 2008

NUTRITIONAL STATUS

Burden of undernutrition (2008)
WHO Child Growth Standards

Stunted (under-fives, 000):	1,880	Underweight (under-fives, 000):	1,370
Share of developing world stunting burden (%):	1.0	Wasted (under-fives, 000):	495
Stunting country rank:	18	Severely wasted (under-fives, 000):	134

Current nutritional status
Percentage of children < 5 years old suffering from:

Stunting: 41 (WHO Child Growth Standards), 32 (NCHS reference population)
Underweight: 30 (WHO Child Growth Standards), 32 (NCHS reference population)
Wasting: 11 (WHO Child Growth Standards), 9 (NCHS reference population)

■ WHO Child Growth Standards
■ NCHS reference population

Source: MICS 2003

Stunting trends
Percentage of children < 5 years old stunted NCHS reference population

1991 Other NS	1994 Other NS	2000 MICS	2003 MICS
48	53	34	32

Underweight trends
Percentage of children < 5 years old underweight NCHS reference population

Insufficient progress towards MDG1

1991 Other NS	1994 Other NS	1995 MICS	1997 MICS	2000 MICS	2003 MICS
41	35	43	39	35	32

INFANT AND YOUNG CHILD FEEDING

Child feeding practices, by age

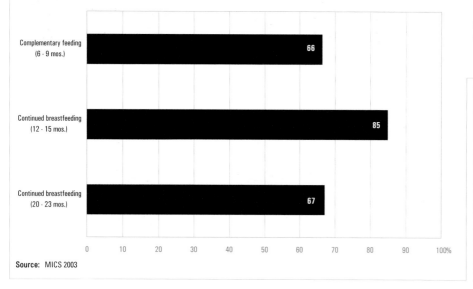

Complementary feeding (6 - 9 mos.): 66
Continued breastfeeding (12 - 15 mos.): 85
Continued breastfeeding (20 - 23 mos.): 67

Source: MICS 2003

Data not available to produce infant feeding practices area graph

Exclusive breastfeeding
Percentage of infants < 6 months old exclusively breastfed

2003 MICS
15

MICRONUTRIENTS

Vitamin A supplementation
Percentage of children 6-59 months old receiving two doses of vitamin A during calendar year

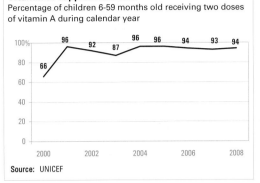

Source: UNICEF

Iodized salt consumption trends*
Percentage of households consuming adequately iodized salt
72,000 newborns are unprotected against IDD (2008)

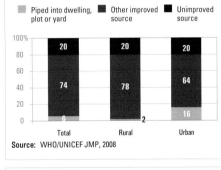

* Estimates may not be comparable.

Anaemia
Prevalence of anaemia among selected population

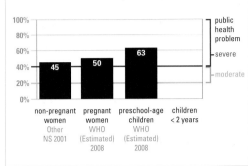

ESSENTIAL NUTRITION INTERVENTIONS DURING THE LIFE CYCLE

Pregnancy	Birth	0-5 months	6-23 months	24-59 months

Use of iron-folic acid supplements	-	Early initiation of breastfeeding (within 1 hour of birth)	-

International Code of Marketing of Breastmilk Substitutes	No
Maternity protection in accordance with ILO Convention 183	No

Household consumption of adequately iodized salt	93%	Infants not weighed at birth	-	Exclusive breastfeeding (<6 months)	15%

Timely introduction of complementary foods (with continued breastfeeding)	66%
Continued breastfeeding at two years	67%

To increase children's chances of survival, improve development and prevent stunting, nutrition interventions need to be delivered during the mother's pregnancy and the first two years of the child's life.

Full coverage of vitamin A supplementation	94%
National guidelines for management of severe acute malnutrition incorporating the community-based approach	Yes
Policy on new ORS formula and zinc for management of diarrhoea	Yes
Policy on community treatment of pneumonia with antibiotics	Yes

MATERNAL NUTRITION/HEALTH

Maternal mortality ratio, adjusted (per 100,000 live births)	380	(2005)
Maternal mortality ratio, reported (per 100,000 live births)	320	(2004-2005)
Total number of maternal deaths	3,700	(2005)
Lifetime risk of maternal death (1 in :)	110	(2005)
Women with low BMI (<18.5 kg/m², %)	-	-
Anaemia, non-pregnant women (<120 g/l, %)	45	(2001)
Antenatal care (at least one visit, %)	76	(2001)
Antenatal care (at least four visits, %)	22	(2001)
Skilled attendant at birth (%)	57	(2001)
Low birthweight (<2,500 grams, %)	15	(2000)
Primary school net enrolment or attendance ratio (% female, % male)	84, 83	(2003)
Gender parity index (primary school net enrolment or attendance ratio)	1.01	(2003)

WATER AND SANITATION

Drinking water coverage
Percentage of population by type of drinking water source, 2006

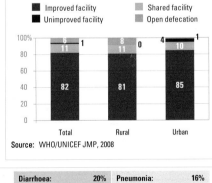

Source: WHO/UNICEF JMP, 2008

Sanitation coverage
Percentage of population by type of sanitation facility, 2006

Source: WHO/UNICEF JMP, 2008

Under-five deaths (post-neonatal) caused by: Diarrhoea: 20% Pneumonia: 16%

DISPARITIES IN NUTRITION

Indicator	Gender			Residence			Wealth quintile						Source
	Male	Female	Ratio of male to female	Urban	Rural	Ratio of urban to rural	Poorest	Second	Middle	Fourth	Richest	Ratio of richest to poorest	
Stunting prevalence (WHO Child Growth Standards, %)	42	40	1.1	32	43	0.7	-	-	-	-	-	-	MICS 2003
Underweight prevalence (WHO Child Growth Standards, %)	31	28	1.1	25	31	0.8	-	-	-	-	-	-	MICS 2003
Wasting prevalence (WHO Child Growth Standards, %)	12	10	1.2	9	11	0.8	-	-	-	-	-	-	MICS 2003
Infants not weighed at birth (%)	-	-	-	-	-	-	-	-	-	-	-	-	-
Early initiation of breastfeeding (%)	-	-	-	-	-	-	-	-	-	-	-	-	-
Women with low BMI (<18.5 kg/m², %)	-	-	-	-	-	-	-	-	-	-	-	-	-

DEMOGRAPHICS

Total population (000)	28,810	(2008)
Total under-five population (000)	3,535	(2008)
Total number of births (000)	732	(2008)
Under-five mortality rate (per 1,000 live births)	51	(2008)
Total number of under-five deaths (000)	37	(2008)
Infant mortality rate (per 1,000 live births)	41	(2008)
Neonatal mortality rate (per 1,000 live births)	32	(2004)
HIV prevalence rate (15–49 years, %)	0.5	(2007)
Population below international poverty line of US$1.25 per day (%)	55	(2003-2004)

Under-five mortality rate
Deaths per 1,000 live births

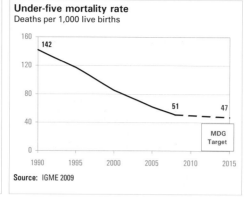

Source: IGME 2009

Causes of under-five deaths, 2004

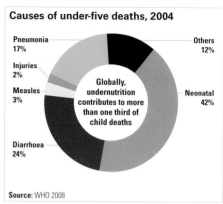

Pneumonia 17%
Others 12%
Injuries 2%
Measles 3%
Neonatal 42%
Diarrhoea 24%

Globally, undernutrition contributes to more than one third of child deaths

Source: WHO 2008

NUTRITIONAL STATUS

Burden of undernutrition (2008)
WHO Child Growth Standards

Stunted (under-fives, 000):	1,743		Underweight (under-fives, 000):	1,365
Share of developing world stunting burden (%):	0.9		Wasted (under-fives, 000):	445
Stunting country rank:	19		Severely wasted (under-fives, 000):	92

Current nutritional status
Percentage of children < 5 years old suffering from:

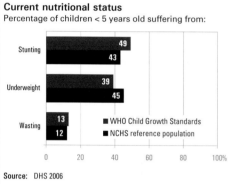

Stunting 49 / 43
Underweight 39 / 45
Wasting 13 / 12

■ WHO Child Growth Standards
■ NCHS reference population

Source: DHS 2006

Stunting trends
Percentage of children < 5 years old stunted NCHS reference population

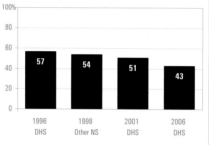

1996 DHS	1998 Other NS	2001 DHS	2006 DHS
57	54	51	43

Underweight trends
Percentage of children < 5 years old underweight NCHS reference population

No progress towards MDG 1

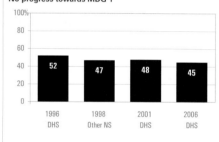

1996 DHS	1998 Other NS	2001 DHS	2006 DHS
52	47	48	45

INFANT AND YOUNG CHILD FEEDING

Infant feeding practices, by age

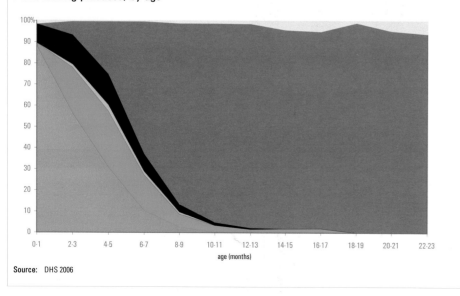

age (months)

Source: DHS 2006

■ Weaned (not breastfed)
■ Breastfed and solid/ semi-solid foods
■ Breastfed and other milk/formula
■ Breastfed and non-milk liquids
■ Breastfed and plain water only
■ Exclusively breastfed

Exclusive breastfeeding
Percentage of infants < 6 months old exclusively breastfed

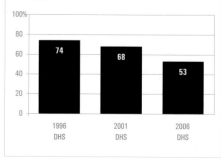

1996 DHS	2001 DHS	2006 DHS
74	68	53

MICRONUTRIENTS

Vitamin A supplementation
Percentage of children 6-59 months old receiving two doses of vitamin A during calendar year

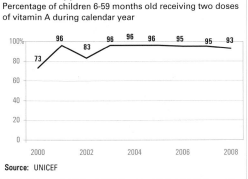

Source: UNICEF

Iodized salt consumption trends*
Percentage of households consuming adequately iodized salt
274,000 newborns are unprotected against IDD (2008)

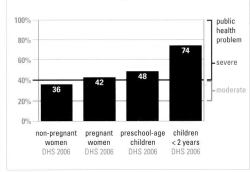

	1995 MICS	1998 Other NS	2000 Other NS
	68	55	63

* Estimates may not be comparable.

Anaemia
Prevalence of anaemia among selected population

non-pregnant women DHS 2006	pregnant women DHS 2006	preschool-age children DHS 2006	children < 2 years DHS 2006
36	42	48	74

public health problem / severe / moderate

ESSENTIAL NUTRITION INTERVENTIONS DURING THE LIFE CYCLE

Pregnancy	Birth	0-5 months	6-23 months	24-59 months

Use of iron-folic acid supplements	7%	Early initiation of breastfeeding (within 1 hour of birth)	35%
Household consumption of adequately iodized salt	63%	Infants not weighed at birth	83%

International Code of Marketing of Breastmilk Substitutes	Yes
Maternity protection in accordance with ILO Convention 183	No
Exclusive breastfeeding (<6 months)	53%

Timely introduction of complementary foods (with continued breastfeeding)	75%
Continued breastfeeding at two years	95%
Full coverage of vitamin A supplementation	93%
National guidelines for management of severe acute malnutrition incorporating the community-based approach	Partial
Policy on new ORS formula and zinc for management of diarrhoea	Yes
Policy on community treatment of pneumonia with antibiotics	Yes

To increase children's chances of survival, improve development and prevent stunting, nutrition interventions need to be delivered during the mother's pregnancy and the first two years of the child's life.

MATERNAL NUTRITION/HEALTH

Maternal mortality ratio, adjusted (per 100,000 live births)	830	(2005)
Maternal mortality ratio, reported (per 100,000 live births)	280	(1999-2005)
Total number of maternal deaths	6,500	(2005)
Lifetime risk of maternal death (1 in :)	31	(2005)
Women with low BMI (<18.5 kg/m², %)	24	(2006)
Anaemia, non-pregnant women (<120 g/l, %)	36	(2006)
Antenatal care (at least one visit, %)	44	(2006)
Antenatal care (at least four visits, %)	29	(2006)
Skilled attendant at birth (%)	19	(2006)
Low birthweight (<2,500 grams, %)	21	(2006)
Primary school net enrolment or attendance ratio (% female, % male)	82, 86	(2006)
Gender parity index (primary school net enrolment or attendance ratio)	0.95	(2006)

WATER AND SANITATION

Drinking water coverage
Percentage of population by type of drinking water source, 2006

Piped into dwelling, plot or yard / Other improved source / Unimproved source

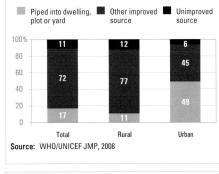

	Total	Rural	Urban
Unimproved source	11	12	6
Other improved source	72	77	45
Piped into dwelling, plot or yard	17	11	49

Source: WHO/UNICEF JMP, 2008

Sanitation coverage
Percentage of population by type of sanitation facility, 2006

Improved facility / Shared facility / Unimproved facility / Open defecation

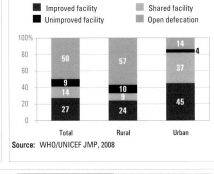

	Total	Rural	Urban
Open defecation	50	57	14
			4
Shared facility	9	10	37
Unimproved facility	14	9	
Improved facility	27	24	45

Source: WHO/UNICEF JMP, 2008

Under-five deaths (post-neonatal) caused by:	Diarrhoea:	24%	Pneumonia:	17%

DISPARITIES IN NUTRITION

Indicator	Gender			Residence			Wealth quintile						Source
	Male	Female	Ratio of male to female	Urban	Rural	Ratio of urban to rural	Poorest	Second	Middle	Fourth	Richest	Ratio of richest to poorest	
Stunting prevalence (WHO Child Growth Standards, %)	49	50	1.0	36	51	0.7	62	55	50	40	31	0.5	DHS 2006
Underweight prevalence (WHO Child Growth Standards, %)	38	40	1.0	23	41	0.6	47	46	42	31	19	0.4	DHS 2006
Wasting prevalence (WHO Child Growth Standards, %)	13	12	1.1	8	13	0.6	12	15	15	13	7	0.6	DHS 2006
Infants not weighed at birth (%)	-	-	-	54	87	0.6	96	91	89	78	46	0.5	DHS 2006
Early initiation of breastfeeding (%)	36	35	1.0	39	35	1.1	30	38	35	35	41	1.4	DHS 2006
Women with low BMI (<18.5 kg/m², %)	-	24	-	17	26	0.7	25	33	29	24	13	0.5	DHS 2006

NIGER

Total population (000)	14,704	(2008)
Total under-five population (000)	3,121	(2008)
Total number of births (000)	791	(2008)
Under-five mortality rate (per 1,000 live births)	167	(2008)
Total number of under-five deaths (000)	121	(2008)
Infant mortality rate (per 1,000 live births)	79	(2008)
Neonatal mortality rate (per 1,000 live births)	41	(2004)
HIV prevalence rate (15–49 years, %)	0.8	(2007)
Population below international poverty line of US$1.25 per day (%)	66	(2005)

Under-five mortality rate
Deaths per 1,000 live births

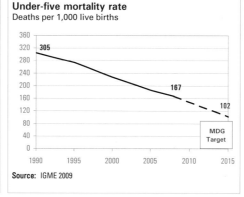

Source: IGME 2009

Causes of under-five deaths, 2004

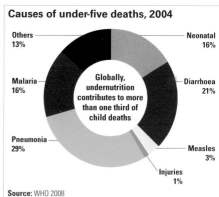

Globally, undernutrition contributes to more than one third of child deaths

- Others 13%
- Neonatal 16%
- Malaria 16%
- Diarrhoea 21%
- Pneumonia 29%
- Measles 3%
- Injuries 1%

Source: WHO 2008

NUTRITIONAL STATUS

Burden of undernutrition (2008)
WHO Child Growth Standards

Stunted (under-fives, 000):	1,473	Underweight (under-fives, 000):	1,108
Share of developing world stunting burden (%):	0.8	Wasted (under-fives, 000):	362
Stunting country rank:	23	Severely wasted (under-fives, 000):	87

Current nutritional status
Percentage of children < 5 years old suffering from:

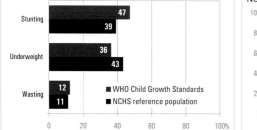

- Stunting: 47 (WHO Child Growth Standards), 39 (NCHS reference population)
- Underweight: 36 (WHO Child Growth Standards), 43 (NCHS reference population)
- Wasting: 12 (WHO Child Growth Standards), 11 (NCHS reference population)

■ WHO Child Growth Standards
■ NCHS reference population

Source: Other NS 2008

Stunting trends
Percentage of children < 5 years old stunted NCHS reference population

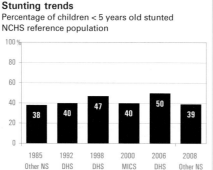

1985 Other NS	1992 DHS	1998 DHS	2000 MICS	2006 DHS	2008 Other NS
38	40	47	40	50	39

Underweight trends
Percentage of children < 5 years old underweight NCHS reference population

No progress towards MDG1

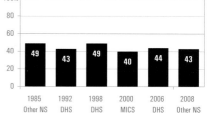

1985 Other NS	1992 DHS	1998 DHS	2000 MICS	2006 DHS	2008 Other NS
49	43	49	40	44	43

INFANT AND YOUNG CHILD FEEDING

Infant feeding practices, by age

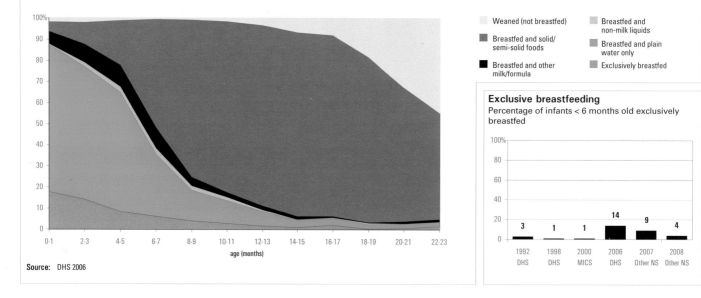

age (months)

- Weaned (not breastfed)
- Breastfed and solid/semi-solid foods
- Breastfed and other milk/formula
- Breastfed and non-milk liquids
- Breastfed and plain water only
- Exclusively breastfed

Source: DHS 2006

Exclusive breastfeeding
Percentage of infants < 6 months old exclusively breastfed

1992 DHS	1998 DHS	2000 MICS	2006 DHS	2007 Other NS	2008 Other NS
3	1	1	14	9	4

MICRONUTRIENTS

Vitamin A supplementation
Percentage of children 6-59 months old receiving two doses of vitamin A during calendar year

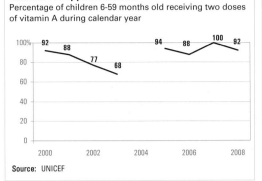

Source: UNICEF

Iodized salt consumption trends*
Percentage of households consuming adequately iodized salt
427,000 newborns are unprotected against IDD (2008)

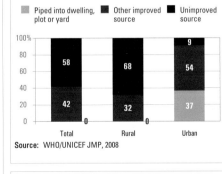

* Estimates may not be comparable.

Anaemia
Prevalence of anaemia among selected population

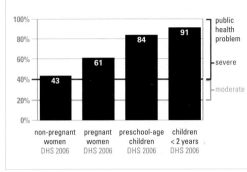

ESSENTIAL NUTRITION INTERVENTIONS DURING THE LIFE CYCLE

Pregnancy	Birth	0-5 months	6-23 months	24-59 months

Use of iron-folic acid supplements	14%	Early initiation of breastfeeding (within 1 hour of birth)	38%

International Code of Marketing of Breastmilk Substitutes	Partial
Maternity protection in accordance with ILO Convention 183	No

Household consumption of adequately iodized salt	46%	Infants not weighed at birth	79%

Exclusive breastfeeding (<6 months)	4%

Timely introduction of complementary foods (with continued breastfeeding)	66%
Continued breastfeeding at two years	-
Full coverage of vitamin A supplementation	92%
National guidelines for management of severe acute malnutrition incorporating the community-based approach	Yes
Policy on new ORS formula and zinc for management of diarrhoea	Yes
Policy on community treatment of pneumonia with antibiotics	Yes

To increase children's chances of survival, improve development and prevent stunting, nutrition interventions need to be delivered during the mother's pregnancy and the first two years of the child's life.

MATERNAL NUTRITION/HEALTH

Maternal mortality ratio, adjusted (per 100,000 live births)	1,800	(2005)
Maternal mortality ratio, reported (per 100,000 live births)	650	(1996-2006)
Total number of maternal deaths	14,000	(2005)
Lifetime risk of maternal death (1 in :)	7	(2005)
Women with low BMI (<18.5 kg/m², %)	19	(2006)
Anaemia, non-pregnant women (<120 g/l, %)	43	(2006)
Antenatal care (at least one visit, %)	46	(2006)
Antenatal care (at least four visits, %)	15	(2006)
Skilled attendant at birth (%)	33	(2006)
Low birthweight (<2,500 grams, %)	27	(2006)
Primary school net enrolment or attendance ratio (% female, % male)	31, 44	(2006)
Gender parity index (primary school net enrolment or attendance ratio)	0.7	(2006)

WATER AND SANITATION

Drinking water coverage
Percentage of population by type of drinking water source, 2006

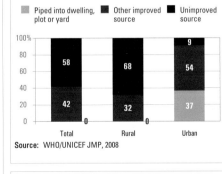

Source: WHO/UNICEF JMP, 2008

Sanitation coverage
Percentage of population by type of sanitation facility, 2006

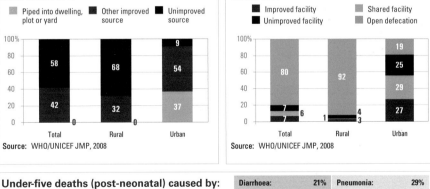

Source: WHO/UNICEF JMP, 2008

Under-five deaths (post-neonatal) caused by:	Diarrhoea:	21%	Pneumonia:	29%

DISPARITIES IN NUTRITION

Indicator	Gender			Residence			Wealth quintile						Source
	Male	Female	Ratio of male to female	Urban	Rural	Ratio of urban to rural	Poorest	Second	Middle	Fourth	Richest	Ratio of richest to poorest	
Stunting prevalence (WHO Child Growth Standards, %)	58	52	1.1	35	58	0.6	57	58	58	59	40	0.7	DHS 2006
Underweight prevalence (WHO Child Growth Standards, %)	41	37	1.1	23	41	0.6	42	42	42	41	25	0.6	DHS 2006
Wasting prevalence (WHO Child Growth Standards, %)	14	12	1.2	10	14	0.7	15	14	15	11	10	0.7	DHS 2006
Infants not weighed at birth (%)	-	-	-	24	89	0.3	92	88	89	84	37	0.4	DHS 2006
Early initiation of breastfeeding (%)	49	48	1.0	62	46	1.3	44	45	45	49	59	1.3	DHS 2006
Women with low BMI (<18.5 kg/m², %)	-	19	-	13	21	0.6	19	20	24	21	13	0.7	DHS 2006

NIGERIA

DEMOGRAPHICS

Total population (000)	151,212	(2008)
Total under-five population (000)	25,020	(2008)
Total number of births (000)	6,028	(2008)
Under-five mortality rate (per 1,000 live births)	186	(2008)
Total number of under-five deaths (000)	1,077	(2008)
Infant mortality rate (per 1,000 live births)	96	(2008)
Neonatal mortality rate (per 1,000 live births)	47	(2004)
HIV prevalence rate (15–49 years, %)	3.1	(2007)
Population below international poverty line of US$1.25 per day (%)	64	(2003-2004)

Under-five mortality rate
Deaths per 1,000 live births

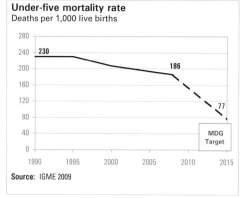

Source: IGME 2009

Causes of under-five deaths, 2004

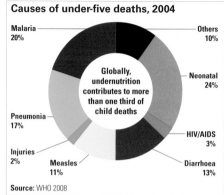

Malaria 20%
Others 10%
Neonatal 24%
HIV/AIDS 3%
Diarrhoea 13%
Measles 11%
Injuries 2%
Pneumonia 17%

Globally, undernutrition contributes to more than one third of child deaths

Source: WHO 2008

NUTRITIONAL STATUS

Burden of undernutrition (2008)
WHO Child Growth Standards

Stunted (under-fives, 000):	10,158	Underweight (under-fives, 000):	5,780
Share of developing world stunting burden (%):	5.2	Wasted (under-fives, 000):	3,478
Stunting country rank:	3	Severely wasted (under-fives, 000):	1,751

Current nutritional status
Percentage of children < 5 years old suffering from:

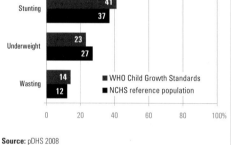

Stunting: 41 / 37
Underweight: 23 / 27
Wasting: 14 / 12

■ WHO Child Growth Standards
■ NCHS reference population

Source: pDHS 2008

Stunting trends
Percentage of children < 5 years old stunted NCHS reference population

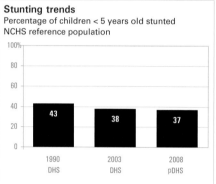

1990 DHS	2003 DHS	2008 pDHS
43	38	37

Underweight trends
Percentage of children < 5 years old underweight NCHS reference population

Insufficient progress towards MDG1

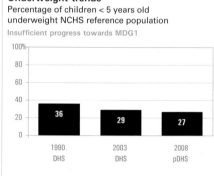

1990 DHS	2003 DHS	2008 pDHS
36	29	27

INFANT AND YOUNG CHILD FEEDING

Infant feeding practices, by age

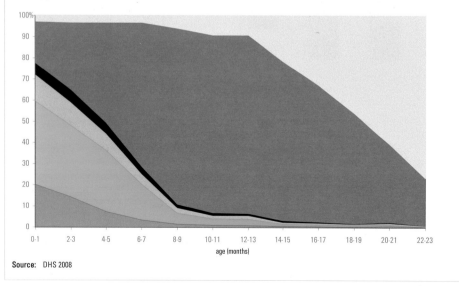

age (months)

Source: DHS 2008

Legend:
- Weaned (not breastfed)
- Breastfed and solid/semi-solid foods
- Breastfed and other milk/formula
- Breastfed and non-milk liquids
- Breastfed and plain water only
- Exclusively breastfed

Exclusive breastfeeding
Percentage of infants < 6 months old exclusively breastfed

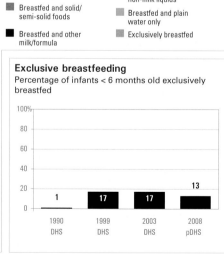

1990 DHS	1999 DHS	2003 DHS	2008 pDHS
1	17	17	13

MICRONUTRIENTS

Vitamin A supplementation
Percentage of children 6-59 months old receiving two doses of vitamin A during calendar year

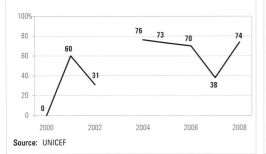

Source: UNICEF

Iodized salt consumption trends*
Percentage of households consuming adequately iodized salt
163,000 newborns are unprotected against IDD (2008)

83	98	97
1995 MICS	1999 DHS	2003 DHS

* Estimates may not be comparable.

Anaemia
Prevalence of anaemia among selected population

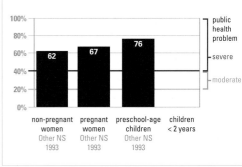

ESSENTIAL NUTRITION INTERVENTIONS DURING THE LIFE CYCLE

Pregnancy	Birth	0-5 months	6-23 months	24-59 months

Use of iron-folic acid supplements	21%	Early initiation of breastfeeding (within 1 hour of birth)	32%	International Code of Marketing of Breastmilk Substitutes — Yes
				Maternity protection in accordance with ILO Convention 183 — No
Household consumption of adequately iodized salt	97%	Infants not weighed at birth	73%	Exclusive breastfeeding (<6 months) 13% — Timely introduction of complementary foods (with continued breastfeeding) 75%

To increase children's chances of survival, improve development and prevent stunting, nutrition interventions need to be delivered during the mother's pregnancy and the first two years of the child's life.

Continued breastfeeding at two years	32%
Full coverage of vitamin A supplementation	74%
National guidelines for management of severe acute malnutrition incorporating the community-based approach	No
Policy on new ORS formula and zinc for management of diarrhoea	Partial
Policy on community treatment of pneumonia with antibiotics	No

MATERNAL NUTRITION/HEALTH

Maternal mortality ratio, adjusted (per 100,000 live births)	1,100	(2005)
Maternal mortality ratio, reported (per 100,000 live births)	-	-
Total number of maternal deaths	59,000	(2005)
Lifetime risk of maternal death (1 in :)	18	(2005)
Women with low BMI (<18.5 kg/m², %)	15	(2003)
Anaemia, non-pregnant women (<120 g/l, %)	62	(1993)
Antenatal care (at least one visit, %)	58	(2008)
Antenatal care (at least four visits, %)	47	(2003)
Skilled attendant at birth (%)	39	(2008)
Low birthweight (<2,500 grams, %)	14	(2003)
Primary school net enrolment or attendance ratio (% female, % male)	58, 68	(2005)
Gender parity index (primary school net enrolment or attendance ratio)	0.85	(2005)

WATER AND SANITATION

Drinking water coverage
Percentage of population by type of drinking water source, 2006

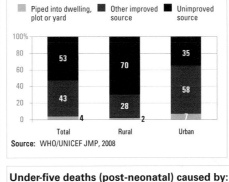

Source: WHO/UNICEF JMP, 2008

Sanitation coverage
Percentage of population by type of sanitation facility, 2006

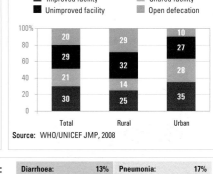

Source: WHO/UNICEF JMP, 2008

Under-five deaths (post-neonatal) caused by: | Diarrhoea: 13% | Pneumonia: 17%

DISPARITIES IN NUTRITION

Indicator	Gender			Residence			Wealth quintile						Source
	Male	Female	Ratio of male to female	Urban	Rural	Ratio of urban to rural	Poorest	Second	Middle	Fourth	Richest	Ratio of richest to poorest	
Stunting prevalence (WHO Child Growth Standards, %)	46	39	1.2	32	47	0.7	54	53	49	36	21	0.4	DHS 2003
Underweight prevalence (WHO Child Growth Standards, %)	29	28	1.0	22	32	0.7	35	38	31	27	13	0.4	DHS 2003
Wasting prevalence (WHO Child Growth Standards, %)	14	13	1.1	11	15	0.7	13	13	10	11	9	0.7	DHS 2003
Infants not weighed at birth (%)	-	-	-	50	82	0.6	91	89	81	63	28	0.3	DHS 2003
Early initiation of breastfeeding (%)	31	33	0.9	35	31	1.1	22	31	37	35	37	1.7	DHS 2003
Women with low BMI (<18.5 kg/m², %)	-	15	-	13	16	0.8	22	18	16	13	9	0.4	DHS 2003

PAKISTAN

Total population (000)	176,952	(2008)
Total under-five population (000)	23,778	(2008)
Total number of births (000)	5,337	(2008)
Under-five mortality rate (per 1,000 live births)	89	(2008)
Total number of under-five deaths (000)	465	(2008)
Infant mortality rate (per 1,000 live births)	72	(2008)
Neonatal mortality rate (per 1,000 live births)	53	(2004)
HIV prevalence rate (15–49 years, %)	0.1	(2007)
Population below international poverty line of US$1.25 per day (%)	23	(2004-2005)

Under-five mortality rate
Deaths per 1,000 live births

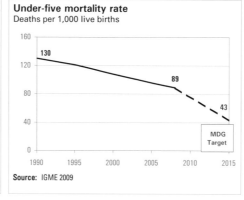

Source: IGME 2009

Causes of under-five deaths, 2004

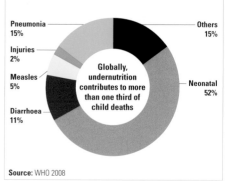

Pneumonia 15%
Injuries 2%
Measles 5%
Diarrhoea 11%
Others 15%
Neonatal 52%

Globally, undernutrition contributes to more than one third of child deaths

Source: WHO 2008

Burden of undernutrition (2008)
WHO Child Growth Standards

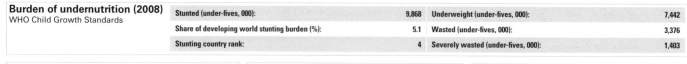

Stunted (under-fives, 000):	9,868	Underweight (under-fives, 000):	7,442
Share of developing world stunting burden (%):	5.1	Wasted (under-fives, 000):	3,376
Stunting country rank:	4	Severely wasted (under-fives, 000):	1,403

Current nutritional status
Percentage of children < 5 years old suffering from:

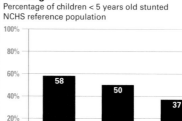

Stunting 42 / 37
Underweight 31 / 38
Wasting 14 / 13

■ WHO Child Growth Standards
■ NCHS reference population

Source: Other NS 2001-2002

Stunting trends
Percentage of children < 5 years old stunted
NCHS reference population

1985 Other NS	1990–1991 DHS	2001–2002 Other NS
58	50	37

Underweight trends
Percentage of children < 5 years old underweight
NCHS reference population
Insufficient progress towards MDG 1

1985 Other NS	1990–1991 DHS	1995 MICS	2001–2002 Other NS
49	40	38	38

Infant feeding practices, by age

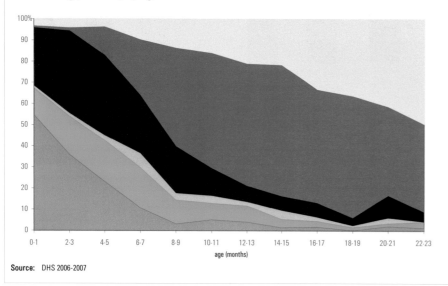

age (months)

Source: DHS 2006-2007

Weaned (not breastfed)
Breastfed and solid/semi-solid foods
Breastfed and other milk/formula
Breastfed and non-milk liquids
Breastfed and plain water only
Exclusively breastfed

Exclusive breastfeeding
Percentage of infants < 6 months old exclusively breastfed

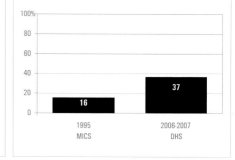

1995 MICS	2006-2007 DHS
16	37

MICRONUTRIENTS

Vitamin A supplementation
Percentage of children 6-59 months old receiving two doses of vitamin A during calendar year

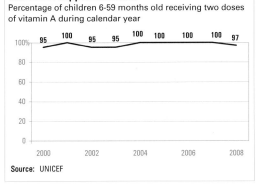

Source: UNICEF

Iodized salt consumption trends*
Percentage of households consuming adequately iodized salt
4,430,000 newborns are unprotected against IDD (2008)

19	17
1995 MICS	2001-2002 Other NS

* Estimates may not be comparable.

Anaemia
Prevalence of anaemia among selected population

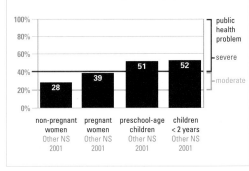

non-pregnant women	pregnant women	preschool-age children	children < 2 years
28	39	51	52
Other NS 2001	Other NS 2001	Other NS 2001	Other NS 2001

public health problem — severe — moderate

ESSENTIAL NUTRITION INTERVENTIONS DURING THE LIFE CYCLE

Pregnancy	Birth	0-5 months	6-23 months	24-59 months

Use of iron-folic acid supplements	16%
Early initiation of breastfeeding (within 1 hour of birth)	29%
International Code of Marketing of Breastmilk Substitutes	Partial
Maternity protection in accordance with ILO Convention 183	No
Household consumption of adequately iodized salt	17%
Infants not weighed at birth	90%
Exclusive breastfeeding (<6 months)	37%
Timely introduction of complementary foods (with continued breastfeeding)	36%
Continued breastfeeding at two years	55%
Full coverage of vitamin A supplementation	97%
National guidelines for management of severe acute malnutrition incorporating the community-based approach	Partial
Policy on new ORS formula and zinc for management of diarrhoea	Yes
Policy on community treatment of pneumonia with antibiotics	Yes

To increase children's chances of survival, improve development and prevent stunting, nutrition interventions need to be delivered during the mother's pregnancy and the first two years of the child's life.

MATERNAL NUTRITION/HEALTH

Maternal mortality ratio, adjusted (per 100,000 live births)	320	(2005)
Maternal mortality ratio, reported (per 100,000 live births)	280	(2006-2007)
Total number of maternal deaths	15,000	(2005)
Lifetime risk of maternal death (1 in :)	74	(2005)
Women with low BMI (<18.5 kg/m², %)	-	-
Anaemia, non-pregnant women (<120 g/l, %)	28	(2001)
Antenatal care (at least one visit, %)	61	(2006-2007)
Antenatal care (at least four visits, %)	28	(2006-2007)
Skilled attendant at birth (%)	39	(2006-2007)
Low birthweight (<2,500 grams, %)	32	(2006-2007)
Primary school net enrolment or attendance ratio (% female, % male)	67, 76	(2006-2007)
Gender parity index (primary school net enrolment or attendance ratio)	0.88	(2006-2007)

WATER AND SANITATION

Drinking water coverage
Percentage of population by type of drinking water source, 2006

■ Piped into dwelling, plot or yard ■ Other improved source ■ Unimproved source

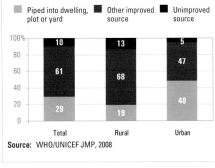

	Total	Rural	Urban
Unimproved	10	13	5
Other improved	61	68	47
Piped	29	19	48

Source: WHO/UNICEF JMP, 2008

Sanitation coverage
Percentage of population by type of sanitation facility, 2006

■ Improved facility ■ Shared facility ■ Unimproved facility ■ Open defecation

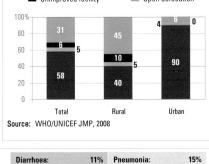

	Total	Rural	Urban
Open defecation	31	45	4 / 6 / 0
	6 / 5	10 / 5	90
Improved	58	40	

Source: WHO/UNICEF JMP, 2008

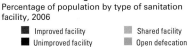
Under-five deaths (post-neonatal) caused by: Diarrhoea: 11% Pneumonia: 15%

DISPARITIES IN NUTRITION

Indicator	Gender			Residence			Wealth quintile						Source
	Male	Female	Ratio of male to female	Urban	Rural	Ratio of urban to rural	Poorest	Second	Middle	Fourth	Richest	Ratio of richest to poorest	
Stunting prevalence (WHO Child Growth Standards, %)	42	41	1.0	36	45	0.8	-	-	-	-	-	-	Other NS 2001-2002
Underweight prevalence (WHO Child Growth Standards, %)	32	31	1.0	29	33	0.9	-	-	-	-	-	-	Other NS 2001-2002
Wasting prevalence (WHO Child Growth Standards, %)	15	13	1.2	14	14	1.0	-	-	-	-	-	-	Other NS 2001-2002
Infants not weighed at birth (%)	-	-	-	78	95	0.8	98	96	92	91	68	0.7	DHS 2006-2007
Early initiation of breastfeeding (%)	28	30	0.9	28	29	1.0	25	28	31	32	30	1.2	DHS 2006-2007
Women with low BMI (<18.5 kg/m², %)	-	-	-	-	-	-	-	-	-	-	-	-	-

DEMOGRAPHICS

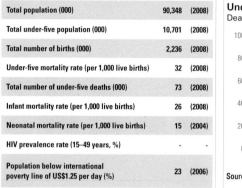

Total population (000)	90,348	(2008)
Total under-five population (000)	10,701	(2008)
Total number of births (000)	2,236	(2008)
Under-five mortality rate (per 1,000 live births)	32	(2008)
Total number of under-five deaths (000)	73	(2008)
Infant mortality rate (per 1,000 live births)	26	(2008)
Neonatal mortality rate (per 1,000 live births)	15	(2004)
HIV prevalence rate (15–49 years, %)	-	-
Population below international poverty line of US$1.25 per day (%)	23	(2006)

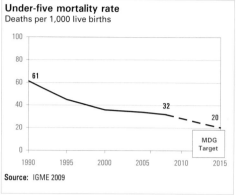

Under-five mortality rate
Deaths per 1,000 live births

Source: IGME 2009

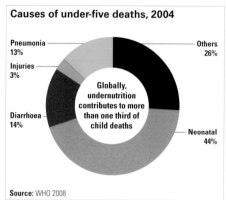

Causes of under-five deaths, 2004

Pneumonia 13%
Injuries 3%
Diarrhoea 14%
Others 26%
Neonatal 44%

Globally, undernutrition contributes to more than one third of child deaths

Source: WHO 2008

NUTRITIONAL STATUS

Burden of undernutrition (2008)
WHO Child Growth Standards

Stunted (under-fives, 000):	3,617	Underweight (under-fives, 000):	2,215
Share of developing world stunting burden (%):	1.9	Wasted (under-fives, 000):	642
Stunting country rank:	9	Severely wasted (under-fives, 000):	171

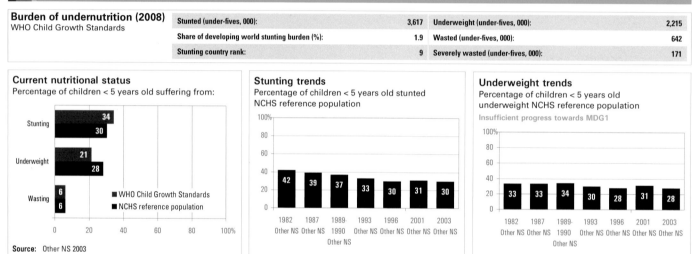

Current nutritional status
Percentage of children < 5 years old suffering from:

Stunting: 34 / 30
Underweight: 21 / 28
Wasting: 6 / 6

■ WHO Child Growth Standards
■ NCHS reference population

Source: Other NS 2003

Stunting trends
Percentage of children < 5 years old stunted
NCHS reference population

1982 Other NS	1987 Other NS	1989-1990 Other NS	1993 Other NS	1996 Other NS	2001 Other NS	2003 Other NS
42	39	37	33	30	31	30

Underweight trends
Percentage of children < 5 years old
underweight NCHS reference population

Insufficient progress towards MDG1

1982 Other NS	1987 Other NS	1989-1990 Other NS	1993 Other NS	1996 Other NS	2001 Other NS	2003 Other NS
33	33	34	30	28	31	28

INFANT AND YOUNG CHILD FEEDING

Infant feeding practices, by age

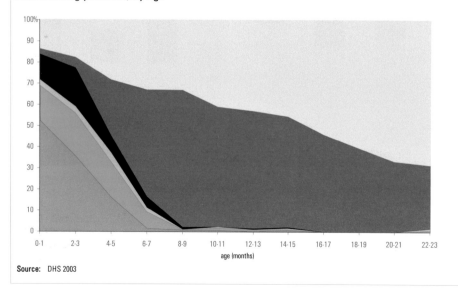

age (months)

Source: DHS 2003

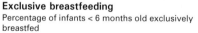

Weaned (not breastfed)
Breastfed and solid/semi-solid foods
Breastfed and other milk/formula
Breastfed and non-milk liquids
Breastfed and plain water only
Exclusively breastfed

Exclusive breastfeeding
Percentage of infants < 6 months old exclusively breastfed

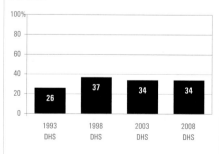

1993 DHS	1998 DHS	2003 DHS	2008 DHS
26	37	34	34

MICRONUTRIENTS

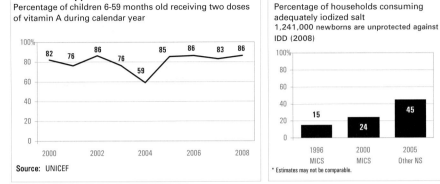

Vitamin A supplementation
Percentage of children 6-59 months old receiving two doses of vitamin A during calendar year

Values: 82 (2000), 76, 86, 76, 59 (2004), 85, 86, 83, 86 (2008)

Source: UNICEF

Iodized salt consumption trends*
Percentage of households consuming adequately iodized salt
1,241,000 newborns are unprotected against IDD (2008)

15 (1996 MICS), 24 (2000 MICS), 45 (2005 Other NS)

* Estimates may not be comparable.

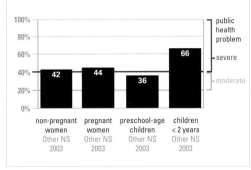

Anaemia
Prevalence of anaemia among selected population

- non-pregnant women (Other NS 2003): 42
- pregnant women (Other NS 2003): 44
- preschool-age children (Other NS 2003): 36
- children < 2 years (Other NS 2003): 66

public health problem — severe — moderate

ESSENTIAL NUTRITION INTERVENTIONS DURING THE LIFE CYCLE

Pregnancy → Birth → 0-5 months → 6-23 months → 24-59 months

Use of iron-folic acid supplements	29%
Household consumption of adequately iodized salt	45%
Early initiation of breastfeeding (within 1 hour of birth)	54%
Infants not weighed at birth	28%
Exclusive breastfeeding (<6 months)	34%
International Code of Marketing of Breastmilk Substitutes	Yes
Maternity protection in accordance with ILO Convention 183	No
Timely introduction of complementary foods (with continued breastfeeding)	58%
Continued breastfeeding at two years	34%
Full coverage of vitamin A supplementation	86%
National guidelines for management of severe acute malnutrition incorporating the community-based approach	Partial
Policy on new ORS formula and zinc for management of diarrhoea	Yes
Policy on community treatment of pneumonia with antibiotics	No

To increase children's chances of survival, improve development and prevent stunting, nutrition interventions need to be delivered during the mother's pregnancy and the first two years of the child's life.

MATERNAL NUTRITION/HEALTH

Indicator	Value	Year
Maternal mortality ratio, adjusted (per 100,000 live births)	230	(2005)
Maternal mortality ratio, reported (per 100,000 live births)	160	(2006)
Total number of maternal deaths	4,600	(2005)
Lifetime risk of maternal death (1 in :)	140	(2005)
Women with low BMI (<18.5 kg/m², %)	-	-
Anaemia, non-pregnant women (<120 g/l, %)	42	(2003)
Antenatal care (at least one visit, %)	91	(2008)
Antenatal care (at least four visits, %)	70	(2003)
Skilled attendant at birth (%)	62	(2008)
Low birthweight (<2,500 grams, %)	20	(2003)
Primary school net enrolment or attendance ratio (% female, % male)	93, 91	(2006)
Gender parity index (primary school net enrolment or attendance ratio)	1.02	(2006)

WATER AND SANITATION

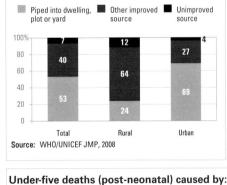

Drinking water coverage
Percentage of population by type of drinking water source, 2006

Legend: Piped into dwelling, plot or yard; Other improved source; Unimproved source

- Total: 53, 40, 7
- Rural: 24, 64, 12
- Urban: 69, 27, 4

Source: WHO/UNICEF JMP, 2008

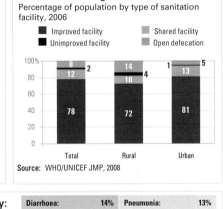

Sanitation coverage
Percentage of population by type of sanitation facility, 2006

Legend: Improved facility; Shared facility; Unimproved facility; Open defecation

- Total: 78, 12, 8, 2
- Rural: 72, 10, 14, 4
- Urban: 81, 13, 1, 5

Source: WHO/UNICEF JMP, 2008

Under-five deaths (post-neonatal) caused by: Diarrhoea: 14%   Pneumonia: 13%

DISPARITIES IN NUTRITION

Indicator	Gender			Residence			Wealth quintile						Source
	Male	Female	Ratio of male to female	Urban	Rural	Ratio of urban to rural	Poorest	Second	Middle	Fourth	Richest	Ratio of richest to poorest	
Stunting prevalence (WHO Child Growth Standards, %)	36	32	1.1	-	-	-	-	-	-	-	-	-	Other NS 2003
Underweight prevalence (WHO Child Growth Standards, %)	20	21	1.0	-	-	-	-	-	-	-	-	-	Other NS 2003
Wasting prevalence (WHO Child Growth Standards, %)	7	6	1.2	-	-	-	-	-	-	-	-	-	Other NS 2003
Infants not weighed at birth (%)	-	-	-	14	41	0.3	51	33	19	11	6	0.1	DHS 2003
Early initiation of breastfeeding (%)	54	55	1.0	54	54	1.0	55	56	53	53	52	0.9	DHS 2003
Women with low BMI (<18.5 kg/m², %)	-	-	-	-	-	-	-	-	-	-	-	-	

SOUTH AFRICA

DEMOGRAPHICS

Total population (000)	49,668	(2008)
Total under-five population (000)	5,200	(2008)
Total number of births (000)	1,091	(2008)
Under-five mortality rate (per 1,000 live births)	67	(2008)
Total number of under-five deaths (000)	73	(2008)
Infant mortality rate (per 1,000 live births)	48	(2008)
Neonatal mortality rate (per 1,000 live births)	17	(2004)
HIV prevalence rate (15–49 years, %)	18.1	(2007)
Population below international poverty line of US$1.25 per day (%)	26	(2000)

Under-five mortality rate
Deaths per 1,000 live births

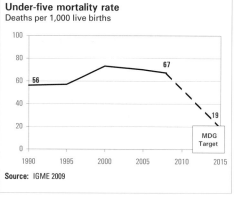

Source: IGME 2009

Causes of under-five deaths, 2004

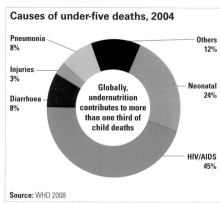

Pneumonia 8%
Injuries 3%
Diarrhoea 8%
Others 12%
Neonatal 24%
HIV/AIDS 45%

Globally, undernutrition contributes to more than one third of child deaths

Source: WHO 2008

NUTRITIONAL STATUS

Burden of undernutrition (2008)
NCHS reference population

Stunted (under-fives, 000):	1,425		Underweight (under-fives, 000):	598
Share of developing world stunting burden (%):	0.7		Wasted (under-fives, 000):	270
Stunting country rank:	24		Severely wasted (under-fives, 000):	94

Current nutritional status
Percentage of children < 5 years old suffering from:

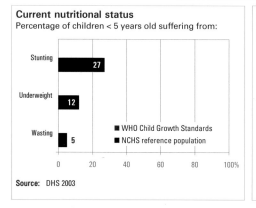

Stunting 27
Underweight 12
Wasting 5

■ WHO Child Growth Standards
■ NCHS reference population

Source: DHS 2003

Stunting trends
Percentage of children < 5 years old stunted
NCHS reference population

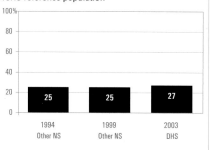

1994 Other NS	1999 Other NS	2003 DHS
25	25	27

Underweight trends
Percentage of children < 5 years old underweight NCHS reference population

No progress towards MDG1

1994 Other NS	1999 Other NS	2003 DHS
9	12	12

INFANT AND YOUNG CHILD FEEDING

Infant feeding practices, by age

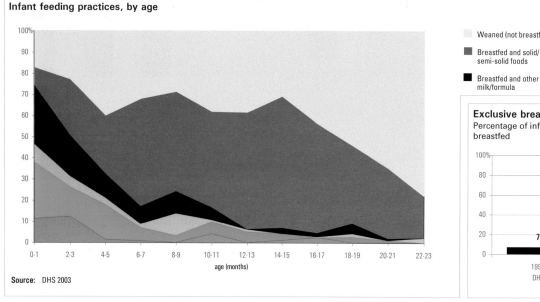

□ Weaned (not breastfed)
■ Breastfed and solid/semi-solid foods
■ Breastfed and other milk/formula
▨ Breastfed and non-milk liquids
▨ Breastfed and plain water only
▨ Exclusively breastfed

Source: DHS 2003

Exclusive breastfeeding
Percentage of infants < 6 months old exclusively breastfed

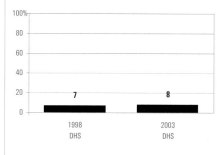

1998 DHS	2003 DHS
7	8

MICRONUTRIENTS

Vitamin A supplementation
Percentage of children 6-59 months old receiving two doses of vitamin A during calendar year

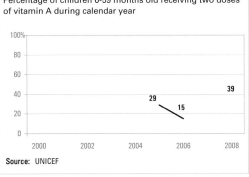

Source: UNICEF

Iodized salt consumption trends*
Percentage of households consuming adequately iodized salt
410,000 newborns are unprotected against IDD (2008)

1998
Other NS

* Estimates may not be comparable.

Anaemia
Prevalence of anaemia among selected population

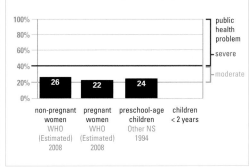

non-pregnant women WHO (Estimated) 2008	26
pregnant women WHO (Estimated) 2008	22
preschool-age children Other NS 1994	24
children < 2 years	

public health problem — severe — moderate

ESSENTIAL NUTRITION INTERVENTIONS DURING THE LIFE CYCLE

Pregnancy ▶ Birth ▶ 0-5 months ▶ 6-23 months ▶ 24-59 months ▶

Use of iron-folic acid supplements	11%
Household consumption of adequately iodized salt	62%

Early initiation of breastfeeding (within 1 hour of birth)	61%
Infants not weighed at birth	32%

International Code of Marketing of Breastmilk Substitutes	Partial
Maternity protection in accordance with ILO Convention 183	No
Exclusive breastfeeding (<6 months)	8%

Timely introduction of complementary foods (with continued breastfeeding)	49%
Continued breastfeeding at two years	31%
Full coverage of vitamin A supplementation	39%
National guidelines for management of severe acute malnutrition incorporating the community-based approach	No
Policy on new ORS formula and zinc for management of diarrhoea	Yes
Policy on community treatment of pneumonia with antibiotics	No

To increase children's chances of survival, improve development and prevent stunting, nutrition interventions need to be delivered during the mother's pregnancy and the first two years of the child's life.

MATERNAL NUTRITION/HEALTH

Maternal mortality ratio, adjusted (per 100,000 live births)	400	(2005)
Maternal mortality ratio, reported (per 100,000 live births)	170	(2003)
Total number of maternal deaths	4,300	(2005)
Lifetime risk of maternal death (1 in :)	110	(2005)
Women with low BMI (<18.5 kg/m², %)	7	(2003)
Anaemia, non-pregnant women (<120 g/l, %)	26	(2008)
Antenatal care (at least one visit, %)	92	(2003)
Antenatal care (at least four visits, %)	56	(2003)
Skilled attendant at birth (%)	91	(2003)
Low birthweight (<2,500 grams, %)	15	(1998)
Primary school net enrolment or attendance ratio (% female, % male)	86, 86	(2005)
Gender parity index (primary school net enrolment or attendance ratio)	1	(2005)

WATER AND SANITATION

Drinking water coverage
Percentage of population by type of drinking water source, 2006

Piped into dwelling, plot or yard ▪ Other improved source ▪ Unimproved source

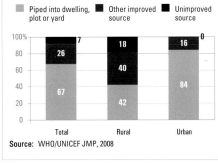

Source: WHO/UNICEF JMP, 2008

Sanitation coverage
Percentage of population by type of sanitation facility, 2006

Improved facility ▪ Shared facility ▪ Unimproved facility ▪ Open defecation

Source: WHO/UNICEF JMP, 2008

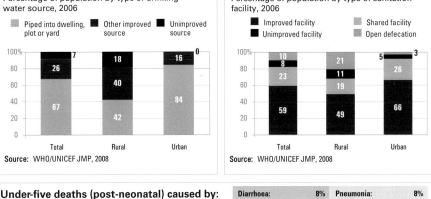

Under-five deaths (post-neonatal) caused by: Diarrhoea: 8%   Pneumonia: 8%

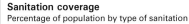

DISPARITIES IN NUTRITION

Indicator	Gender			Residence			Wealth quintile						Source
	Male	Female	Ratio of male to female	Urban	Rural	Ratio of urban to rural	Poorest	Second	Middle	Fourth	Richest	Ratio of richest to poorest	
Stunting prevalence (NCHS reference population, %)	28	27	1.0	27	28	1.0	-	-	-	-	-	-	DHS 2003
Underweight prevalence (NCHS reference population, %)	13	11	1.2	12	11	1.1	-	-	-	-	-	-	DHS 2003
Wasting prevalence (NCHS reference population, %)	7	4	1.8	6	5	1.2	-	-	-	-	-	-	DHS 2003
Infants not weighed at birth (%)	-	-	-	26	38	0.7	-	-	-	-	-	-	DHS 1998
Early initiation of breastfeeding (%)	62	61	1.0	61	62	1.0	-	-	-	-	-	-	DHS 2003
Women with low BMI (<18.5 kg/m², %)	-	7	-	6	7	0.9	-	-	-	-	-	-	DHS 2003

SUDAN

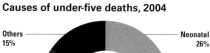

DEMOGRAPHICS

Total population (000)	41,348	(2008)
Total under-five population (000)	5,836	(2008)
Total number of births (000)	1,296	(2008)
Under-five mortality rate (per 1,000 live births)	109	(2008)
Total number of under-five deaths (000)	138	(2008)
Infant mortality rate (per 1,000 live births)	70	(2008)
Neonatal mortality rate (per 1,000 live births)	27	(2004)
HIV prevalence rate (15–49 years, %)	1.4	(2007)
Population below international poverty line of US$1.25 per day (%)	-	

Under-five mortality rate
Deaths per 1,000 live births

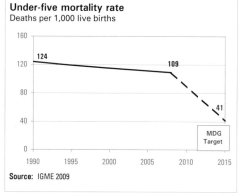

Source: IGME 2009

Causes of under-five deaths, 2004

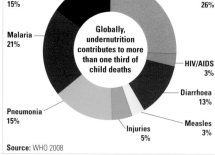

Globally, undernutrition contributes to more than one third of child deaths

- Others 15%
- Neonatal 26%
- Malaria 21%
- HIV/AIDS 3%
- Diarrhoea 13%
- Measles 3%
- Injuries 5%
- Pneumonia 15%

Source: WHO 2008

NUTRITIONAL STATUS

Burden of undernutrition (2008)
WHO Child Growth Standards

Stunted (under-fives, 000):	2,305	Underweight (under-fives, 000):	1,576
Share of developing world stunting burden (%):	1.2	Wasted (under-fives, 000):	945
Stunting country rank:	15	Severely wasted (under-fives, 000):	403

Current nutritional status
Percentage of children < 5 years old suffering from:

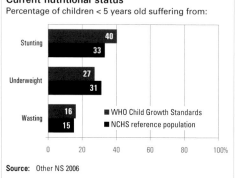

- Stunting: 40 / 33
- Underweight: 27 / 31
- Wasting: 16 / 15

■ WHO Child Growth Standards
■ NCHS reference population

Source: Other NS 2006

Stunting trends
Percentage of children < 5 years old stunted
NCHS reference population

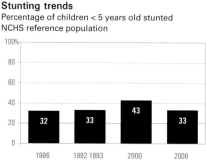

1986 Other NS	1992-1993 Other NS	2000 MICS	2006 Other NS
32	33	43	33

Underweight trends
Percentage of children < 5 years old
underweight NCHS reference population

Insufficient progress towards MDG1

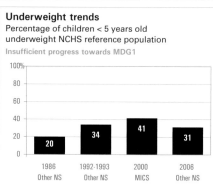

1986 Other NS	1992-1993 Other NS	2000 MICS	2006 Other NS
20	34	41	31

INFANT AND YOUNG CHILD FEEDING

Infant feeding practices, by age

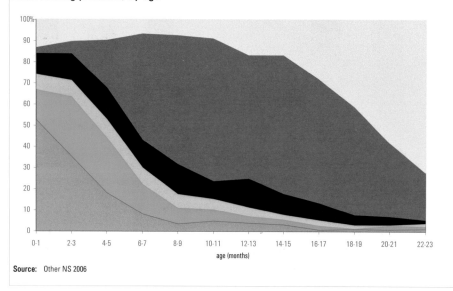

age (months)

- Weaned (not breastfed)
- Breastfed and non-milk liquids
- Breastfed and solid/semi-solid foods
- Breastfed and plain water only
- Breastfed and other milk/formula
- Exclusively breastfed

Source: Other NS 2006

Exclusive breastfeeding
Percentage of infants < 6 months old exclusively breastfed

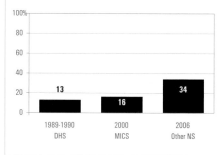

1989-1990 DHS	2000 MICS	2006 Other NS
13	16	34

MICRONUTRIENTS

Vitamin A supplementation
Percentage of children 6-59 months old receiving two doses of vitamin A during calendar year

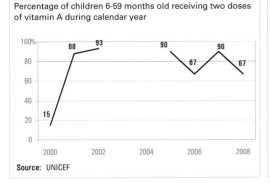

Source: UNICEF

Iodized salt consumption trends*
Percentage of households consuming adequately iodized salt
1,153,000 newborns are unprotected against IDD (2008)

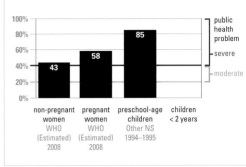

* Estimates may not be comparable.

Anaemia
Prevalence of anaemia among selected population

ESSENTIAL NUTRITION INTERVENTIONS DURING THE LIFE CYCLE

| Pregnancy | Birth | 0-5 months | 6-23 months | 24-59 months |

Use of iron-folic acid supplements	-	Early initiation of breastfeeding (within 1 hour of birth)	-
		International Code of Marketing of Breastmilk Substitutes	Partial
		Maternity protection in accordance with ILO Convention 183	No
Household consumption of adequately iodized salt	11%	Infants not weighed at birth	-
		Exclusive breastfeeding (<6 months)	34%
		Timely introduction of complementary foods (with continued breastfeeding)	56%
		Continued breastfeeding at two years	35%
		Full coverage of vitamin A supplementation	67%
		National guidelines for management of severe acute malnutrition incorporating the community-based approach	Partial
		Policy on new ORS formula and zinc for management of diarrhoea	Partial
		Policy on community treatment of pneumonia with antibiotics	Yes

To increase children's chances of survival, improve development and prevent stunting, nutrition interventions need to be delivered during the mother's pregnancy and the first two years of the child's life.

MATERNAL NUTRITION/HEALTH

Maternal mortality ratio, adjusted (per 100,000 live births)	450	(2005)
Maternal mortality ratio, reported (per 100,000 live births)	1,100	(2006)
Total number of maternal deaths	5,300	(2005)
Lifetime risk of maternal death (1 in :)	53	(2005)
Women with low BMI (<18.5 kg/m², %)	-	-
Anaemia, non-pregnant women (<120 g/l, %)	43	(2008)
Antenatal care (at least one visit, %)	64	(2006)
Antenatal care (at least four visits, %)	-	-
Skilled attendant at birth (%)	49	(2006)
Low birthweight (<2,500 grams, %)	31	(1999)
Primary school net enrolment or attendance ratio (% female, % male)	52, 56	(2006)
Gender parity index (primary school net enrolment or attendance ratio)	0.93	(2006)

WATER AND SANITATION

Drinking water coverage
Percentage of population by type of drinking water source, 2006

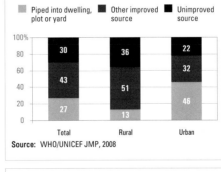

Source: WHO/UNICEF JMP, 2008

Sanitation coverage
Percentage of population by type of sanitation facility, 2006

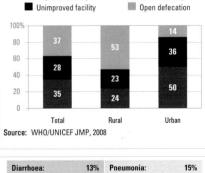

Source: WHO/UNICEF JMP, 2008

Under-five deaths (post-neonatal) caused by: Diarrhoea: 13% Pneumonia: 15%

DISPARITIES IN NUTRITION

Indicator	Gender			Residence			Wealth quintile						Source
	Male	Female	Ratio of male to female	Urban	Rural	Ratio of urban to rural	Poorest	Second	Middle	Fourth	Richest	Ratio of richest to poorest	
Stunting prevalence (WHO Child Growth Standards, %)	42	37	1.1	35	42	0.8	39	45	44	39	28	0.7	Other NS 2006
Underweight prevalence (WHO Child Growth Standards, %)	28	26	1.1	21	30	0.7	31	33	30	23	17	0.5	Other NS 2006
Wasting prevalence (WHO Child Growth Standards, %)	17	15	1.1	14	18	0.8	24	20	15	12	11	0.5	Other NS 2006
Infants not weighed at birth (%)	-	-	-	-	-	-	-	-	-	-	-	-	-
Early initiation of breastfeeding (%)	-	-	-	-	-	-	-	-	-	-	-	-	-
Women with low BMI (<18.5 kg/m², %)	-	-	-	-	-	-	-	-	-	-	-	-	-

UGANDA

DEMOGRAPHICS

Total population (000)	31,657	(2008)
Total under-five population (000)	6,182	(2008)
Total number of births (000)	1,466	(2008)
Under-five mortality rate (per 1,000 live births)	135	(2008)
Total number of under-five deaths (000)	190	(2008)
Infant mortality rate (per 1,000 live births)	85	(2008)
Neonatal mortality rate (per 1,000 live births)	30	(2004)
HIV prevalence rate (15–49 years, %)	5.4	(2007)
Population below international poverty line of US$1.25 per day (%)	52	(2005)

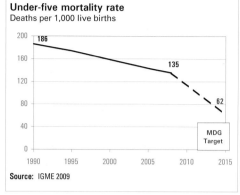

Under-five mortality rate
Deaths per 1,000 live births

Source: IGME 2009

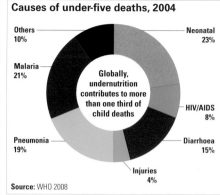

Causes of under-five deaths, 2004

Others 10%
Neonatal 23%
Malaria 21%
HIV/AIDS 8%
Pneumonia 19%
Diarrhoea 15%
Injuries 4%

Globally, undernutrition contributes to more than one third of child deaths

Source: WHO 2008

NUTRITIONAL STATUS

Burden of undernutrition (2008)
WHO Child Growth Standards

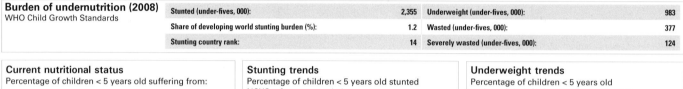

Stunted (under-fives, 000):	2,355		Underweight (under-fives, 000):	983
Share of developing world stunting burden (%):	1.2		Wasted (under-fives, 000):	377
Stunting country rank:	14		Severely wasted (under-fives, 000):	124

Current nutritional status
Percentage of children < 5 years old suffering from:

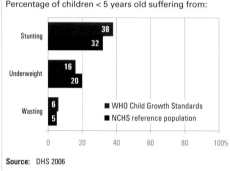

Stunting 38 / 32
Underweight 16 / 20
Wasting 6 / 5

■ WHO Child Growth Standards
■ NCHS reference population

Source: DHS 2006

Stunting trends
Percentage of children < 5 years old stunted
NCHS reference population

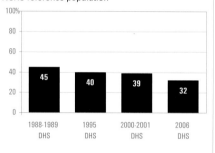

1988-1989 DHS	1995 DHS	2000-2001 DHS	2006 DHS
45	40	39	32

Underweight trends
Percentage of children < 5 years old
underweight NCHS reference population

Insufficient progress towards MDG1

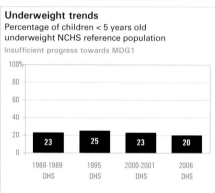

1988-1989 DHS	1995 DHS	2000-2001 DHS	2006 DHS
23	25	23	20

INFANT AND YOUNG CHILD FEEDING

Infant feeding practices, by age

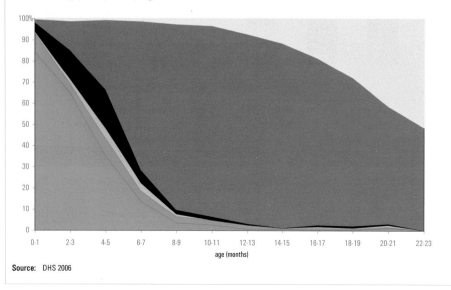

age (months)

Source: DHS 2006

Weaned (not breastfed)
Breastfed and solid/semi-solid foods
Breastfed and other milk/formula
Breastfed and non-milk liquids
Breastfed and plain water only
Exclusively breastfed

Exclusive breastfeeding
Percentage of infants < 6 months old exclusively breastfed

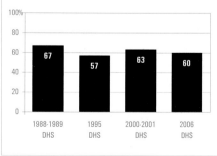

1988-1989 DHS	1995 DHS	2000-2001 DHS	2006 DHS
67	57	63	60

MICRONUTRIENTS

Vitamin A supplementation
Percentage of children 6-59 months old receiving two doses of vitamin A during calendar year

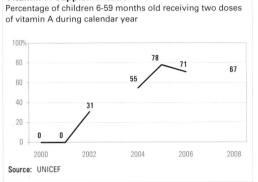

Source: UNICEF

Iodized salt consumption trends*
Percentage of households consuming adequately iodized salt
62,000 newborns are unprotected against IDD (2008)

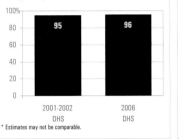

* Estimates may not be comparable.

Anaemia
Prevalence of anaemia among selected population

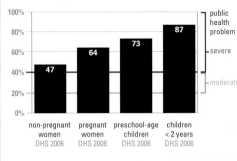

ESSENTIAL NUTRITION INTERVENTIONS DURING THE LIFE CYCLE

Pregnancy	Birth	0-5 months	6-23 months	24-59 months

Use of iron-folic acid supplements	1%	
Household consumption of adequately iodized salt	96%	

Early initiation of breastfeeding (within 1 hour of birth)	42%
Infants not weighed at birth	65%

International Code of Marketing of Breastmilk Substitutes	Yes
Maternity protection in accordance with ILO Convention 183	No
Exclusive breastfeeding (<6 months)	60%

Timely introduction of complementary foods (with continued breastfeeding)	80%
Continued breastfeeding at two years	54%
Full coverage of vitamin A supplementation	67%
National guidelines for management of severe acute malnutrition incorporating the community-based approach	Yes
Policy on new ORS formula and zinc for management of diarrhoea	Partial
Policy on community treatment of pneumonia with antibiotics	Partial

To increase children's chances of survival, improve development and prevent stunting, nutrition interventions need to be delivered during the mother's pregnancy and the first two years of the child's life.

MATERNAL NUTRITION/HEALTH

Maternal mortality ratio, adjusted (per 100,000 live births)	550	(2005)
Maternal mortality ratio, reported (per 100,000 live births)	440	(1997-2006)
Total number of maternal deaths	8,100	(2005)
Lifetime risk of maternal death (1 in :)	25	(2005)
Women with low BMI (<18.5 kg/m², %)	12	(2006)
Anaemia, non-pregnant women (<120 g/l, %)	47	(2006)
Antenatal care (at least one visit, %)	94	(2006)
Antenatal care (at least four visits, %)	47	(2006)
Skilled attendant at birth (%)	42	(2006)
Low birthweight (<2,500 grams, %)	14	(2006)
Primary school net enrolment or attendance ratio (% female, % male)	82, 83	(2006)
Gender parity index (primary school net enrolment or attendance ratio)	0.99	(2006)

WATER AND SANITATION

Drinking water coverage
Percentage of population by type of drinking water source, 2006

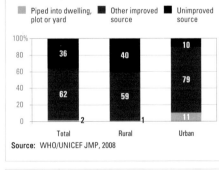

Source: WHO/UNICEF JMP, 2008

Sanitation coverage
Percentage of population by type of sanitation facility, 2006

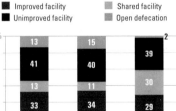

Source: WHO/UNICEF JMP, 2008

Under-five deaths (post-neonatal) caused by:	Diarrhoea:	15%	Pneumonia:	19%

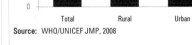

DISPARITIES IN NUTRITION

Indicator	Gender			Residence			Wealth quintile						Source
	Male	Female	Ratio of male to female	Urban	Rural	Ratio of urban to rural	Poorest	Second	Middle	Fourth	Richest	Ratio of richest to poorest	
Stunting prevalence (WHO Child Growth Standards, %)	41	36	1.1	26	40	0.7	43	38	44	38	24	0.6	DHS 2006
Underweight prevalence (WHO Child Growth Standards, %)	17	14	1.2	11	17	0.6	21	16	17	17	8	0.4	DHS 2006
Wasting prevalence (WHO Child Growth Standards, %)	7	5	1.4	7	6	1.2	6	6	7	6	6	1.0	DHS 2006
Infants not weighed at birth (%)	-	-	-	27	70	0.4	73	75	74	62	33	0.5	DHS 2006
Early initiation of breastfeeding (%)	41	43	1.0	48	41	1.2	42	42	39	41	47	1.1	DHS 2006
Women with low BMI (<18.5 kg/m², %)	-	12	-	6	14	0.4	23	15	12	9	6	0.3	DHS 2006

UNITED REPUBLIC OF TANZANIA

DEMOGRAPHICS

Total population (000)	42,484	(2008)
Total under-five population (000)	7,566	(2008)
Total number of births (000)	1,771	(2008)
Under-five mortality rate (per 1,000 live births)	104	(2008)
Total number of under-five deaths (000)	175	(2008)
Infant mortality rate (per 1,000 live births)	67	(2008)
Neonatal mortality rate (per 1,000 live births)	35	(2004)
HIV prevalence rate (15–49 years, %)	6.2	(2007)
Population below international poverty line of US$1.25 per day (%)	89	(2000-2001)

Under-five mortality rate
Deaths per 1,000 live births

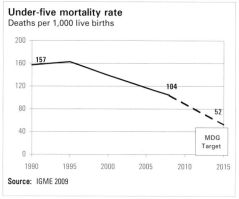

Source: IGME 2009

Causes of under-five deaths, 2004

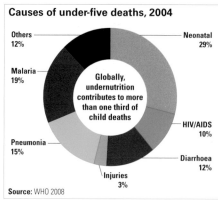

Globally, undernutrition contributes to more than one third of child deaths

Others 12%
Neonatal 29%
Malaria 19%
HIV/AIDS 10%
Pneumonia 15%
Diarrhoea 12%
Injuries 3%

Source: WHO 2008

NUTRITIONAL STATUS

Burden of undernutrition (2008)
WHO Child Growth Standards

Stunted (under-fives, 000):	3,359	Underweight (under-fives, 000):	1,263
Share of developing world stunting burden (%):	1.7	Wasted (under-fives, 000):	265
Stunting country rank:	10	Severely wasted (under-fives, 000):	76

Current nutritional status
Percentage of children < 5 years old suffering from:

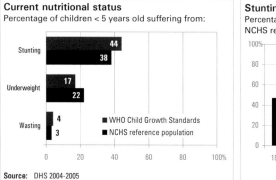

Stunting 44 / 38
Underweight 17 / 22
Wasting 4 / 3

■ WHO Child Growth Standards
■ NCHS reference population

Source: DHS 2004-2005

Stunting trends
Percentage of children < 5 years old stunted
NCHS reference population

47	43	44	38
1991-1992 DHS	1996 DHS	1999 DHS	2004-2005 DHS

Underweight trends
Percentage of children < 5 years old
underweight NCHS reference population
Insufficient progress towards MDG1

29	31	29	22
1991-1992 DHS	1996 DHS	1999 DHS	2004-2005 DHS

INFANT AND YOUNG CHILD FEEDING

Infant feeding practices, by age

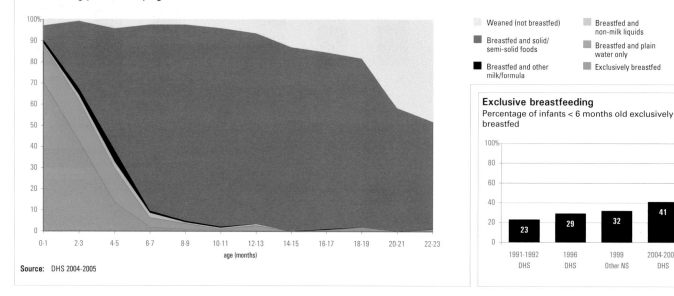

age (months)

Source: DHS 2004-2005

□ Weaned (not breastfed)
■ Breastfed and solid/semi-solid foods
■ Breastfed and other milk/formula
□ Breastfed and non-milk liquids
■ Breastfed and plain water only
■ Exclusively breastfed

Exclusive breastfeeding
Percentage of infants < 6 months old exclusively breastfed

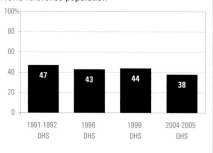

23	29	32	41
1991-1992 DHS	1996 DHS	1999 Other NS	2004-2005 DHS

MICRONUTRIENTS

Vitamin A supplementation
Percentage of children 6-59 months old receiving two doses of vitamin A during calendar year

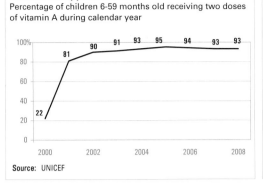

Source: UNICEF

Iodized salt consumption trends*
Percentage of households consuming adequately iodized salt
1,003,000 newborns are unprotected against IDD (2008)

* Estimates may not be comparable.

Anaemia
Prevalence of anaemia among selected population

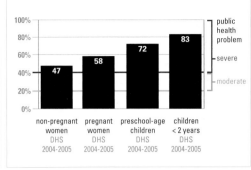

non-pregnant women	pregnant women	preschool-age children	children < 2 years
DHS 2004-2005	DHS 2004-2005	DHS 2004-2005	DHS 2004-2005
47	58	72	83

public health problem — severe — moderate

ESSENTIAL NUTRITION INTERVENTIONS DURING THE LIFE CYCLE

| Pregnancy | Birth | 0-5 months | 6-23 months | 24-59 months |

| Use of iron-folic acid supplements | 10% |
| Household consumption of adequately iodized salt | 43% |

| Early initiation of breastfeeding (within 1 hour of birth) | 67% |
| Infants not weighed at birth | 50% |

International Code of Marketing of Breastmilk Substitutes	Yes
Maternity protection in accordance with ILO Convention 183	No
Exclusive breastfeeding (<6 months)	41%

Timely introduction of complementary foods (with continued breastfeeding)	91%
Continued breastfeeding at two years	55%
Full coverage of vitamin A supplementation	93%
National guidelines for management of severe acute malnutrition incorporating the community-based approach	Yes
Policy on new ORS formula and zinc for management of diarrhoea	Yes
Policy on community treatment of pneumonia with antibiotics	No

To increase children's chances of survival, improve development and prevent stunting, nutrition interventions need to be delivered during the mother's pregnancy and the first two years of the child's life.

MATERNAL NUTRITION/HEALTH

Maternal mortality ratio, adjusted (per 100,000 live births)	950	(2005)
Maternal mortality ratio, reported (per 100,000 live births)	580	(2004-2005)
Total number of maternal deaths	13,000	(2005)
Lifetime risk of maternal death (1 in :)	24	(2005)
Women with low BMI (<18.5 kg/m², %)	10	(2004-2005)
Anaemia, non-pregnant women (<120 g/l, %)	47	(2004-2005)
Antenatal care (at least one visit, %)	76	(2007-2008)
Antenatal care (at least four visits, %)	62	(2004-2005)
Skilled attendant at birth (%)	43	(2004-2005)
Low birthweight (<2,500 grams, %)	10	(2004-2005)
Primary school net enrolment or attendance ratio (% female, % male)	75, 71	(2004-2005)
Gender parity index (primary school net enrolment or attendance ratio)	1.06	(2004-2005)

WATER AND SANITATION

Drinking water coverage
Percentage of population by type of drinking water source, 2006

Piped into dwelling, plot or yard — Other improved source — Unimproved source

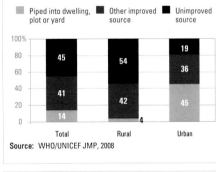

Source: WHO/UNICEF JMP, 2008

Sanitation coverage
Percentage of population by type of sanitation facility, 2006

Improved facility — Shared facility — Unimproved facility — Open defecation

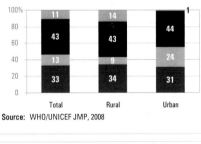

Source: WHO/UNICEF JMP, 2008

Under-five deaths (post-neonatal) caused by: Diarrhoea: 12% Pneumonia: 15%

DISPARITIES IN NUTRITION

Indicator	Gender			Residence			Wealth quintile						Source
	Male	Female	Ratio of male to female	Urban	Rural	Ratio of urban to rural	Poorest	Second	Middle	Fourth	Richest	Ratio of richest to poorest	
Stunting prevalence (WHO Child Growth Standards, %)	47	42	1.1	33	47	0.7	-	-	-	-	-	-	DHS 2004-2005
Underweight prevalence (WHO Child Growth Standards, %)	18	15	1.2	12	18	0.7	-	-	-	-	-	-	DHS 2004-2005
Wasting prevalence (WHO Child Growth Standards, %)	4	3	1.3	3	4	0.8	-	-	-	-	-	-	DHS 2004-2005
Infants not weighed at birth (%)	-	-	-	16	58	0.3	65	59	58	42	10	0.2	DHS 2004-2005
Early initiation of breastfeeding (%)	58	60	1.0	67	58	1.2	54	55	59	62	70	1.3	DHS 2004-2005
Women with low BMI (<18.5 kg/m², %)	-	10	-	8	12	0.7	13	12	11	10	7	0.5	DHS 2004-2005

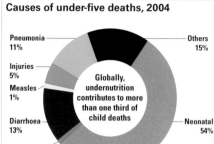

VIET NAM

DEMOGRAPHICS

Total population (000)	87,096	(2008)
Total under-five population (000)	7,316	(2008)
Total number of births (000)	1,494	(2008)
Under-five mortality rate (per 1,000 live births)	14	(2008)
Total number of under-five deaths (000)	21	(2008)
Infant mortality rate (per 1,000 live births)	12	(2008)
Neonatal mortality rate (per 1,000 live births)	12	(2004)
HIV prevalence rate (15–49 years, %)	0.5	(2007)
Population below international poverty line of US$1.25 per day (%)	22	(2006)

Under-five mortality rate
Deaths per 1,000 live births

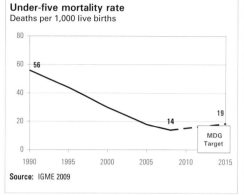

Source: IGME 2009

Causes of under-five deaths, 2004

Pneumonia 11%
Injuries 5%
Measles 1%
Diarrhoea 13%
HIV/AIDS 1%
Others 15%
Neonatal 54%

Globally, undernutrition contributes to more than one third of child deaths

Source: WHO 2008

NUTRITIONAL STATUS

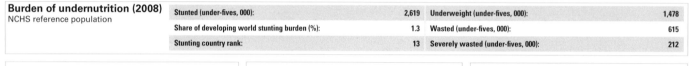

Burden of undernutrition (2008)
NCHS reference population

Stunted (under-fives, 000):	2,619	Underweight (under-fives, 000):	1,478
Share of developing world stunting burden (%):	1.3	Wasted (under-fives, 000):	615
Stunting country rank:	13	Severely wasted (under-fives, 000):	212

Current nutritional status
Percentage of children < 5 years old suffering from:

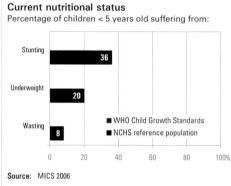

Stunting 36
Underweight 20
Wasting 8

■ WHO Child Growth Standards
■ NCHS reference population

Source: MICS 2006

Stunting trends
Percentage of children < 5 years old stunted NCHS reference population

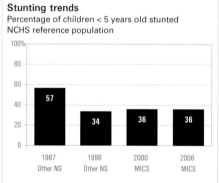

1987 Other NS	1998 Other NS	2000 MICS	2006 MICS
57	34	36	36

Underweight trends
Percentage of children < 5 years old underweight NCHS reference population

On track towards MDG1

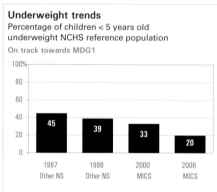

1987 Other NS	1998 Other NS	2000 MICS	2006 MICS
45	39	33	20

INFANT AND YOUNG CHILD FEEDING

Infant feeding practices, by age

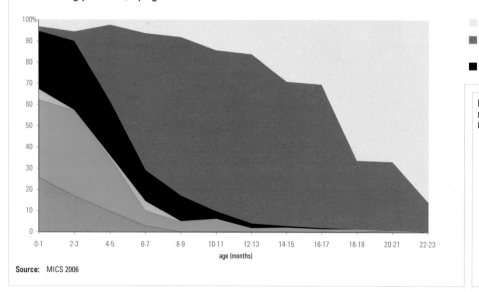

age (months)

Source: MICS 2006

Legend:
- Weaned (not breastfed)
- Breastfed and solid/semi-solid foods
- Breastfed and other milk/formula
- Breastfed and non-milk liquids
- Breastfed and plain water only
- Exclusively breastfed

Exclusive breastfeeding
Percentage of infants < 6 months old exclusively breastfed

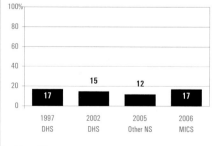

1997 DHS	2002 DHS	2005 Other NS	2006 MICS
17	15	12	17

MICRONUTRIENTS

Vitamin A supplementation
Percentage of children 6-59 months old receiving two doses of vitamin A during calendar year

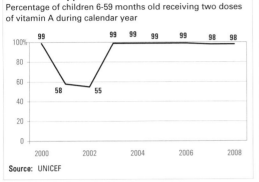

Source: UNICEF

Iodized salt consumption trends*
Percentage of households consuming adequately iodized salt
102,000 newborns are unprotected against IDD (2008)

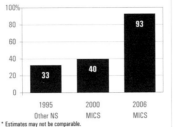

1995 Other NS
2000 MICS
2006 MICS

* Estimates may not be comparable.

Anaemia
Prevalence of anaemia among selected population

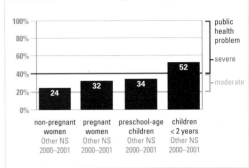

non-pregnant women Other NS 2000–2001	24
pregnant women Other NS 2000–2001	32
preschool-age children Other NS 2000–2001	34
children < 2 years Other NS 2000–2001	52

public health problem — severe — moderate

ESSENTIAL NUTRITION INTERVENTIONS DURING THE LIFE CYCLE

Pregnancy	Birth	0-5 months	6-23 months	24-59 months

Use of iron-folic acid supplements	–	Early initiation of breastfeeding (within 1 hour of birth)	58%	
Household consumption of adequately iodized salt	93%	Infants not weighed at birth	13%	

International Code of Marketing of Breastmilk Substitutes	Partial
Maternity protection in accordance with ILO Convention 183	No

Exclusive breastfeeding (<6 months)	17%	Timely introduction of complementary foods (with continued breastfeeding)	70%
		Continued breastfeeding at two years	23%

Full coverage of vitamin A supplementation	98%
National guidelines for management of severe acute malnutrition incorporating the community-based approach	No
Policy on new ORS formula and zinc for management of diarrhoea	No
Policy on community treatment of pneumonia with antibiotics	Partial

To increase children's chances of survival, improve development and prevent stunting, nutrition interventions need to be delivered during the mother's pregnancy and the first two years of the child's life.

MATERNAL NUTRITION/HEALTH

Maternal mortality ratio, adjusted (per 100,000 live births)	150	(2005)
Maternal mortality ratio, reported (per 100,000 live births)	160	(1994-2006)
Total number of maternal deaths	2,500	(2005)
Lifetime risk of maternal death (1 in :)	280	(2005)
Women with low BMI (<18.5 kg/m², %)	-	-
Anaemia, non-pregnant women (<120 g/l, %)	24	(2000-2001)
Antenatal care (at least one visit, %)	91	(2006)
Antenatal care (at least four visits, %)	29	(2002)
Skilled attendant at birth (%)	88	(2006)
Low birthweight (<2,500 grams, %)	7	(2006)
Primary school net enrolment or attendance ratio (% female, % male)	91, 96	(2001)
Gender parity index (primary school net enrolment or attendance ratio)	0.95	(2001)

WATER AND SANITATION

Drinking water coverage
Percentage of population by type of drinking water source, 2006

Piped into dwelling, plot or yard | Other improved source | Unimproved source

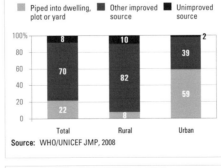

Source: WHO/UNICEF JMP, 2008

Sanitation coverage
Percentage of population by type of sanitation facility, 2006

Improved facility | Shared facility
Unimproved facility | Open defecation

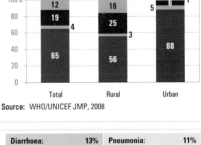

Source: WHO/UNICEF JMP, 2008

Under-five deaths (post-neonatal) caused by:	Diarrhoea:	13%	Pneumonia:	11%

DISPARITIES IN NUTRITION

Indicator	Gender			Residence			Wealth quintile						Source
	Male	Female	Ratio of male to female	Urban	Rural	Ratio of urban to rural	Poorest	Second	Middle	Fourth	Richest	Ratio of richest to poorest	
Stunting prevalence (NCHS reference population, %)	40	32	1.3	24	39	0.6	46	42	32	33	21	0.5	MICS 2006
Underweight prevalence (NCHS reference population, %)	21	19	1.1	12	22	0.5	29	25	17	16	10	0.3	MICS 2006
Wasting prevalence (NCHS reference population, %)	9	8	1.2	9	8	1.1	10	8	10	7	7	0.7	MICS 2006
Infants not weighed at birth (%)	-	-	-	0	17	-	-	-	-	-	-	-	MICS 2006
Early initiation of breastfeeding (%)	-	-	-	54	59	0.9	-	-	-	-	-	-	MICS 2006
Women with low BMI (<18.5 kg/m², %)	-	-	-	-	-	-	-	-	-	-	-	-	-

YEMEN

Total population (000)	22,917	(2008)
Total under-five population (000)	3,733	(2008)
Total number of births (000)	846	(2008)
Under-five mortality rate (per 1,000 live births)	69	(2008)
Total number of under-five deaths (000)	57	(2008)
Infant mortality rate (per 1,000 live births)	53	(2008)
Neonatal mortality rate (per 1,000 live births)	41	(2004)
HIV prevalence rate (15–49 years, %)	-	-
Population below international poverty line of US$1.25 per day (%)	18	(2005)

Under-five mortality rate
Deaths per 1,000 live births

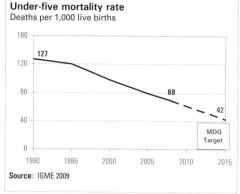

Source: IGME 2009

Causes of under-five deaths, 2004

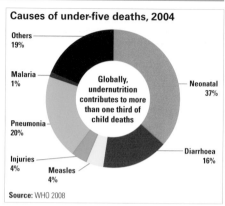

Others 19%
Malaria 1%
Pneumonia 20%
Injuries 4%
Measles 4%
Neonatal 37%
Diarrhoea 16%

Globally, undernutrition contributes to more than one third of child deaths

Source: WHO 2008

Burden of undernutrition (2008)
WHO Child Growth Standards

Stunted (under-fives, 000):	2,154	Underweight (under-fives, 000):	1,609
Share of developing world stunting burden (%):	1.1	Wasted (under-fives, 000):	567
Stunting country rank:	17	Severely wasted (under-fives, 000):	235

Current nutritional status
Percentage of children < 5 years old suffering from:

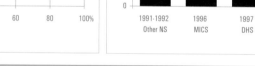

Stunting 58 / 53
Underweight 43 / 46
Wasting 15 / 12

■ WHO Child Growth Standards
■ NCHS reference population

Source: Other NS 2003

Stunting trends
Percentage of children < 5 years old stunted NCHS reference population

1991-1992 Other NS	1996 MICS	1997 DHS	2003 Other NS
44	39	52	53

Underweight trends
Percentage of children < 5 years old underweight NCHS reference population

No progress towards MDG1

1991-1992 Other NS	1996 MICS	1997 DHS	2003 Other NS
30	39	46	46

Infant feeding practices, by age

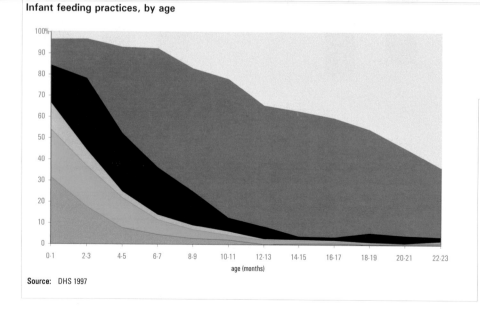

age (months)

Weaned (not breastfed)
Breastfed and solid/semi-solid foods
Breastfed and other milk/formula
Breastfed and non-milk liquids
Breastfed and plain water only
Exclusively breastfed

Source: DHS 1997

Exclusive breastfeeding
Percentage of infants < 6 months old exclusively breastfed

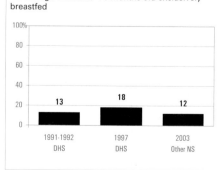

1991-1992 DHS	1997 DHS	2003 Other NS
13	18	12

MICRONUTRIENTS

Vitamin A supplementation
Percentage of children 6-59 months old receiving two doses of vitamin A during calendar year

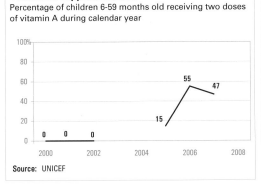

Source: UNICEF

Iodized salt consumption trends*
Percentage of households consuming adequately iodized salt
596,000 newborns are unprotected against IDD (2008)

	1996 MICS	1997 DHS	2003 Other NS
	21	39	30

* Estimates may not be comparable.

Anaemia
Prevalence of anaemia among selected population

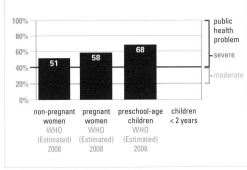

ESSENTIAL NUTRITION INTERVENTIONS DURING THE LIFE CYCLE

Pregnancy	Birth	0-5 months	6-23 months	24-59 months

Use of iron-folic acid supplements	-	Early initiation of breastfeeding (within 1 hour of birth)	30%
Household consumption of adequately iodized salt	30%	Infants not weighed at birth	92%

International Code of Marketing of Breastmilk Substitutes	Yes
Maternity protection in accordance with ILO Convention 183	No
Exclusive breastfeeding (<6 months)	12%

Timely introduction of complementary foods (with continued breastfeeding)	76%
Continued breastfeeding at two years	-
Full coverage of vitamin A supplementation	-
National guidelines for management of severe acute malnutrition incorporating the community-based approach	Yes
Policy on new ORS formula and zinc for management of diarrhoea	Yes
Policy on community treatment of pneumonia with antibiotics	No

To increase children's chances of survival, improve development and prevent stunting, nutrition interventions need to be delivered during the mother's pregnancy and the first two years of the child's life.

MATERNAL NUTRITION/HEALTH

Maternal mortality ratio, adjusted (per 100,000 live births)	430	(2005)
Maternal mortality ratio, reported (per 100,000 live births)	370	(2002-2003)
Total number of maternal deaths	3,600	(2005)
Lifetime risk of maternal death (1 in :)	39	(2005)
Women with low BMI (<18.5 kg/m², %)	25	(1997)
Anaemia, non-pregnant women (<120 g/l, %)	51	(2008)
Antenatal care (at least one visit, %)	47	(2006)
Antenatal care (at least four visits, %)	11	(1997)
Skilled attendant at birth (%)	36	(2006)
Low birthweight (<2,500 grams, %)	32	(1997)
Primary school net enrolment or attendance ratio (% female, % male)	64, 75	(2006)
Gender parity index (primary school net enrolment or attendance ratio)	0.85	(2006)

WATER AND SANITATION

Drinking water coverage
Percentage of population by type of drinking water source, 2006

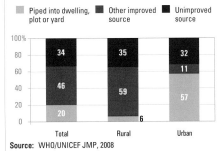

Source: WHO/UNICEF JMP, 2008

Sanitation coverage
Percentage of population by type of sanitation facility, 2006

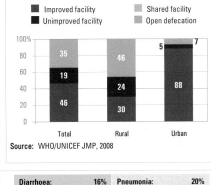

Source: WHO/UNICEF JMP, 2008

Under-five deaths (post-neonatal) caused by: Diarrhoea: 16%   Pneumonia: 20%

DISPARITIES IN NUTRITION

Indicator	Gender			Residence			Wealth quintile						Source
	Male	Female	Ratio of male to female	Urban	Rural	Ratio of urban to rural	Poorest	Second	Middle	Fourth	Richest	Ratio of richest to poorest	
Stunting prevalence (WHO Child Growth Standards, %)	-	-	-	-	-	-	-	-	-	-	-	-	
Underweight prevalence (NCHS reference population, %)	46	45	1.0	37	48	0.8	-	-	-	-	-	-	Other NS 2003
Wasting prevalence (WHO Child Growth Standards, %)	-	-	-	-	-	-	-	-	-	-	-	-	
Infants not weighed at birth (%)	-	-	-	77	96	0.8	-	-	-	-	-	-	DHS 1997
Early initiation of breastfeeding (%)	47	48	1.0	55	45	1.2	-	-	-	-	-	-	DHS 1997
Women with low BMI (<18.5 kg/m², %)	-	25	-	16	28	0.6	-	-	-	-	-	-	DHS 1997

INTERPRETING INFANT AND YOUNG CHILD FEEDING AREA GRAPHS

The infant feeding practices area graphs that appear in the country nutrition profiles offer a snapshot of data on breastfeeding and infant feeding practices as captured by the MICS, DHS, or other surveys. These graphs highlight the status of infant feeding in a country, how close or far it is from the 'ideal', and what some of the major problems may be.

The area graphs are color coded. Ideally, the graphs should be pink before 6 months old, which indicates that all children are exclusively breastfed, and then grey until 24 months, which is an indication that child feeding is optimal among young children.

The 2006 graph for Uganda *(Figure 1)* has a very large pink area at the youngest ages, indicating that a large proportion of children under 6 months old are exclusively breastfed. The large grey area after 6 months old indicates that a substantial proportion of children receive both breastmilk and complementary foods as recommended.

To improve feeding patterns in Uganda, exclusive breastfeeding until an infant is 6 months old can be further increased if the introduction of milks and other liquids is delayed (indicated by lavender and two shades of blue).

The 2006 graph for Niger *(Figure 2)* indicates that although most children receive breastmilk during their first 6 months, very few are breastfed exclusively (almost no pink area).

To increase the exclusive breastfeeding rate, programmes can discourage feeding of plain water to children under 6 months old (bright blue portion of the graph) and discourage introduction of solid or semi-solid foods before 6 months of age (grey).

All available country area graphs can be found at: <www.childinfo.org/breastfeeding_infantfeeding>.

Figure 1. Breastfeeding practices by age, Uganda, 2006

Infant feeding practices, by age

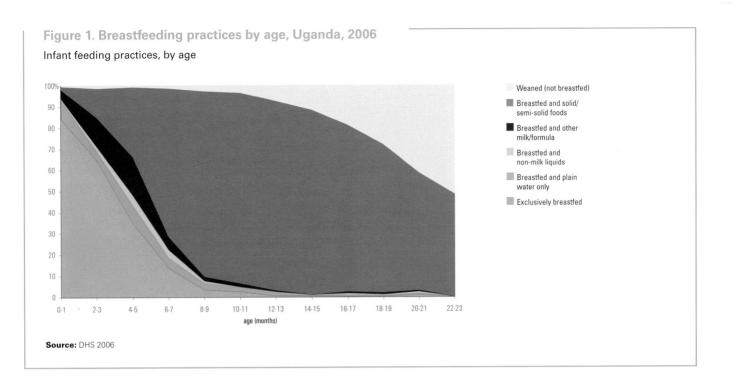

Legend:
- Weaned (not breastfed)
- Breastfed and solid/semi-solid foods
- Breastfed and other milk/formula
- Breastfed and non-milk liquids
- Breastfed and plain water only
- Exclusively breastfed

age (months)

Source: DHS 2006

Figure 2. Breastfeeding practices by age, Niger, 2006

Infant feeding practices, by age

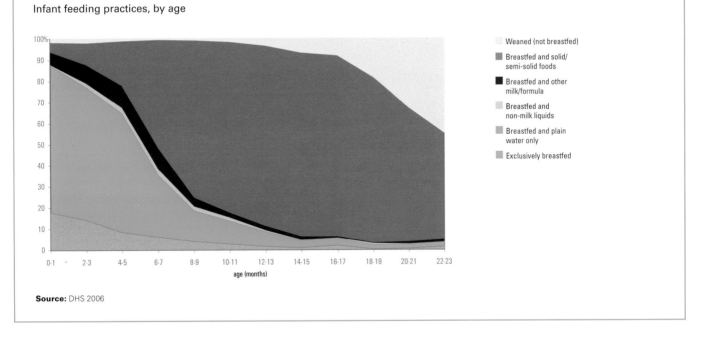

Legend:
- Weaned (not breastfed)
- Breastfed and solid/semi-solid foods
- Breastfed and other milk/formula
- Breastfed and non-milk liquids
- Breastfed and plain water only
- Exclusively breastfed

age (months)

Source: DHS 2006

DATA SOURCES

Indicator		Data source	Global database
Demographics			
General	Total population	United Nations Population Division	United Nations Population Division
	Total under-five population	United Nations Population Division	United Nations Population Division
	Total number of births	United Nations Population Division	United Nations Population Division
Child mortality	Under-five mortality rate	Inter-agency Group for Child Mortality Estimation (IGME) United Nations Children's Fund, World Health Organization, World Bank, United Nations Population Division	Inter-agency Group for Child Mortality Estimation (IGME) United Nations Children's Fund, World Health Organization, World Bank, United Nations Population Division
	Total number of under-five deaths	Inter-agency Group for Child Mortality Estimation (IGME) United Nations Children's Fund, World Health Organization, World Bank, United Nations Population Division	Inter-agency Group for Child Mortality Estimation (IGME) United Nations Children's Fund, World Health Organization, World Bank, United Nations Population Division
	Causes of under-five deaths	World Health Organization, The Global Burden of Disease, 2004 Update (2008)	World Health Organization
	Infant mortality rate	Inter-agency Group for Child Mortality Estimation (IGME) United Nations Children's Fund, World Health Organization, World Bank, United Nations Population Division	Inter-agency Group for Child Mortality Estimation (IGME) United Nations Children's Fund, World Health Organization, World Bank, United Nations Population Division
	Neonatal mortality rate	World Health Organization	World Health Organization
HIV and AIDS	HIV prevalence rate (15–49 years old)	*Report on the Global AIDS Epidemic*, 2008	Joint United Nations Programme on HIV/AIDS (UNAIDS)
Poverty	Population below international poverty line of US$1.25 per day (%)	World Bank	World Bank
Nutritional status			
Anthropometry	Stunting prevalence	Demographic and Health Surveys, Multiple Indicator Cluster Surveys, other national household surveys	United Nations Children's Fund, World Health Organization
	Underweight prevalence	Demographic and Health Surveys, Multiple Indicator Cluster Surveys, other national household surveys	United Nations Children's Fund, World Health Organization
	Wasting prevalence	Demographic and Health Surveys, Multiple Indicator Cluster Surveys, other national household surveys	United Nations Children's Fund, World Health Organization
Infant feeding	Early initiation of breastfeeding (<1 hour)	Demographic and Health Surveys, Multiple Indicator Cluster Surveys	United Nations Children's Fund
	Exclusive breastfeeding rate (<6 months)	Demographic and Health Surveys, Multiple Indicator Cluster Surveys, other national household surveys	United Nations Children's Fund
	Breastfed with complementary food (6–9 months)	Demographic and Health Surveys, Multiple Indicator Cluster Surveys, other national household surveys	United Nations Children's Fund
	Continued breastfeeding at two years (20–23 months)	Demographic and Health Surveys, Multiple Indicator Cluster Surveys, other national household surveys	United Nations Children's Fund
Micronutrients	Vitamin A supplementation (full coverage)	National immunization days reporting, Demographic and Health Surveys, Multiple Indicator Cluster Surveys, routine reporting	United Nations Children's Fund

(continued)

Indicator		Data source	Global database
Nutritional status (continued)			
	Iodized salt consumption	Demographic and Health Surveys, Multiple Indicator Cluster Surveys, other national household surveys	United Nations Children's Fund
	Anaemia prevalence	*Worldwide Prevalence of Anaemia 1993–2005,* WHO Global Database on Anaemia, with additional data from Demographic and Health Surveys and the World Health Organization global database on anaemia	World Health Organization
	Use of iron-folic acid supplements	Demographic and Health Surveys (2003–2008)	N/A
Low birthweight	Low birthweight incidence	Demographic and Health Surveys, Multiple Indicator Cluster Surveys, other national household surveys	United Nations Children's Fund
	Children not weighed at birth	Demographic and Health Surveys, Multiple Indicator Cluster Surveys, other national household surveys	United Nations Children's Fund
Maternal nutrition and health			
Maternal mortality	Maternal mortality ratio (adjusted) *Inter-agency adjusted estimates*	United Nations Children's Fund, World Health Organization, United Nations Population Fund, World Bank	United Nations Children's Fund, World Health Organization, United Nations Population Fund, World Bank
	Maternal mortality ratio (reported) *National authority estimates*	Vital registration systems, routine data reporting, Demographic and Health Surveys, Multiple Indicator Cluster Surveys, and other national household surveys	United Nations Children's Fund
	Total number of maternal deaths	United Nations Children's Fund, World Health Organization, United Nations Population Fund, World Bank	United Nations Children's Fund, World Health Organization, United Nations Population Fund, World Bank
	Lifetime risk of maternal death	United Nations Children's Fund, World Health Organization, United Nations Population Fund, World Bank	United Nations Children's Fund, World Health Organization, United Nations Population Fund, World Bank
Nutrition	Women with low BMI	Demographic and Health Surveys	United Nations Children's Fund
	Anaemia, non-pregnant women	*Worldwide Prevalence of Anaemia 1993–2005,* WHO Global Database on Anaemia; with additional data from Demographic and Health Surveys and the World Health Organization global database on anaemia	World Health Organization
Maternal health	Antenatal care (at least one visit)	Demographic and Health Surveys, Multiple Indicator Cluster Surveys, Reproductive Health Survey, Family Health Survey	United Nations Children's Fund
	Antenatal care (at least four visits)	Demographic and Health Surveys, Multiple Indicator Cluster Surveys, other national household surveys	United Nations Children's Fund, World Health Organization
Delivery care	Skilled attendant at birth	Demographic and Health Surveys, Multiple Indicator Cluster Surveys, other national household surveys	United Nations Children's Fund

Indicator		Data source	Global database
Education			
Education	Primary school net enrolment ratio or net attendance ratio (female, male)	Attendance: Demographic and Health Surveys, Multiple Indicator Cluster Surveys, other surveys Enrolment: UNESCO Institute for Statistics (UIS)	United Nations Children's Fund
	Gender parity index (primary school)	UNESCO Institute for Statistics, Demographic and Health Surveys, Multiple Indicator Cluster Surveys	United Nations Children's Fund
Water and sanitation			
Water	Drinking water coverage	United Nations Children's Fund, World Health Organization	Joint Monitoring Programme for Water Supply and Sanitation – World Health Organization, United Nations Children's Fund
Sanitation	Sanitation coverage	United Nations Children's Fund, World Health Organization	Joint Monitoring Programme for Water Supply and Sanitation – World Health Organization, United Nations Children's Fund
Policies			
Policies	International Code of Marketing of Breastmilk Substitutes	United Nations Children's Fund, World Health Organization	Special data compilation by World Health Organization for Countdown 2008 Report. Updates and information for non-Countdown countries provided by United Nations Children's Fund in August 2009.
	Maternity protection in accordance with International Labour Organization (ILO) Convention no. 183	World Health Organization, United Nations Children's Fund, Zinc Task Force	Special data compilation by World Health Organization for Countdown 2008 Report. Updates and information for non-Countdown countries provided by United Nations Children's Fund in August 2009.
	National guidelines for management of severe acute malnutrition (SAM) incorporating the community-based approach	United Nations Children's Fund, Nutrition Section	Special data compilation by UNICEF for regular programme monitoring. Updated in August 2009.
	New oral rehydration salts (ORS) formula and zinc for management of diarrhoea	ILOLEX (Database of International Labour Standards)	International Labor Organization (2009)
	Community treatment of pneumonia with antibiotics	World Health Organization, United Nations Children's Fund	Special data compilation by World Health Organization for Countdown 2008 Report. Updates and information for non-Countdown countries provided by United Nations Children's Fund in August 2009.

DEFINITIONS OF KEY INDICATORS

Indicator name	Definition	Numerator	Denominator
Demographics			
Under-five mortality rate	Probability of dying between birth and exactly 5 years of age, expressed per 1,000 live births		
Infant mortality rate	Probability of dying between birth and exactly 1 year of age, expressed per 1,000 live births		
Neonatal mortality rate	Probability of dying during the first 28 completed days of life, expressed per 1,000 live births		
HIV prevalence rate (15–49 years old)	Percentage of adults (15–49 years old) living with HIV as of 2007		
Population below international poverty line of US$1.25 per day (%)	Percentage of population living on less than US$1.25 per day at 2005 prices, adjusted for purchasing power parity		
Nutritional status			
Stunting prevalence	Percentage of children under 5 years old who fall below minus two (moderate and severe) and below minus three (severe) standard deviations from median height for age of reference population	Number of children under 5 years old who (a) fall below minus two standard deviations (moderate and severe) (b) fall below minus three standard deviations (severe) from the median height for age of the reference population	Total number of children under 5 years old
Underweight prevalence	Percentage of children under 5 years old who fall below minus two (moderate and severe) and below minus three (severe) standard deviations from median weight for age of reference population	Number of children under 5 years old who (a) fall below minus two standard deviations (moderate and severe) (b) fall below minus three standard deviations (severe) from the median weight for age of the reference population	Total number of children under 5 years old
Wasting prevalence	Percentage of children under 5 years old who fall below minus two (moderate and severe) and below minus three (severe) standard deviations from median weight for height of reference population	Number of children under 5 years old who (a) fall below minus two standard deviations (moderate and severe) (b) fall below minus three standard deviations (severe) from the median weight for height of the reference population	Total number of children under 5 years old
Early initiation of breastfeeding (<1 hour)	Percentage of newborns put to the breast within one hour of birth	Number of women with a live birth during the X years prior to the survey who put the newborn infant to the breast within one hour of birth	Total number of women with a live birth during the same period *(note: this reference period may differ between surveys)*
Exclusive breastfeeding (<6 months)	Percentage of infants 0–5 months old who are exclusively breastfed	Number of infants 0–5 months old who are exclusively breastfed	Total number of infants 0–5 months old
Breastfed with complementary food (6–9 months old)	Percentage of infants 6–9 months old who are breastfed and receive complementary food	Number of infants 6–9 months old who are breastfed and receive complementary food	Total number of infants 6–9 months old
Continued breastfeeding at two years	Percentage of children 20–23 months old who are currently breastfeeding	Number of children 20–23 months old who are currently breastfeeding	Total number of children 20–23 months old
Vitamin A supplementation (full coverage)	Percentage of children 6–59 months old who received two doses during the calendar year *(refer to 'General notes on the data', page 117, for details)*		
Iodized salt consumption	Percentage of households consuming adequately iodized salt	Number of households with salt testing 15 parts per million or more of iodide/iodate	Total number of households

Definitions of key indicators (continued)

Indicator name	Definition	Numerator	Denominator
Child nutrition (continued)			
Anaemia among non-pregnant women	Percentage of non-pregnant women 15–49 years of age with haemoglobin concentration <120 g/L	Number of non-pregnant women 15–49 years old who had a haemoglobin concentration <120 g/L	Total number of non-pregnant women 15–49 years old
Anaemia among pregnant women	Percentage of pregnant women with haemoglobin concentration <110 g/L	Number of pregnant women 15–49 years old who had a haemoglobin concentration <110 g/L	Total number of pregnant women 15–49 years old
Anaemia among pre-school aged children	Percentage of preschool-age* children with haemoglobin concentration <110 g/L *Age range may vary by country*	Number of pre-school aged children who had a haemoglobin concentration <110 g/L	Total number of preschool-age children
Anaemia among children under 2 years old	Percentage of children under 2 years old with haemoglobin concentration <110 g/L (age range may vary by country)	Number of children less than 2 years old who had a haemoglobin concentration <110 g/L	Total number of children under 2 years old
Use of iron-folic acid supplements	Percentage of women who took iron-folic acid supplements for at least 90 days during their last pregnancy in the 5 years prior to the survey	Number of women who took iron-folic acid supplements for at least 90 days during their last pregnancy in the 5 years prior to the survey	Total number of women who had a live birth during the same period
Low birthweight incidence	Percentage of live births that weighed less than 2,500 grams at birth	Number of last live births in the X years prior to the survey weighing below 2,500 grams at birth	Total number of last live births during the same period
Children not weighed at birth	Percentage of live births that were not weighed at birth	Number of last live births in the X years prior to the survey who were not weighed at birth	Total number of last live births during the same period
Maternal nutrition and health			
Maternal mortality ratio	Number of deaths of women from pregnancy-related causes per 100,000 live births		
Lifetime risk of maternal death	Lifetime risk of maternal death takes into account both the probability of becoming pregnant and the probability of dying as a result of that pregnancy accumulated across a woman's reproductive years		
Women with low BMI	Percentage of women 15–49 years old with a body mass index (BMI) of less than 18.5	Number of women 15–49 years old with a BMI <18.5	Total number of women 15–49 years old
Antenatal care (at least one visit)	Percentage of women 15–49 years old attended at least once during pregnancy by skilled health personnel for reasons related to the pregnancy	Number of women attended at least once during pregnancy by skilled health personnel (doctor, nurse, midwife or auxiliary midwife) for reasons related to the pregnancy during the X years prior to the survey	Total number of women who had a live birth occurring in the same period
Antenatal care (at least four visits)	Percentage of women 15–49 years old attended at least four times during pregnancy by any provider (skilled or unskilled) for reasons related to the pregnancy	Number of women attended at least four times during pregnancy by any provider (skilled or unskilled) for reasons related to the pregnancy during the X years prior to the survey	Total number of women who had a live birth occurring in the same period
Skilled attendant at birth	Percentage of live births attended by skilled health personnel	Number of live births to women 15–49 years old in the X years prior to the survey attended during delivery by skilled health personnel (doctor, nurse, midwife or auxiliary midwife)	Total number of live births to women 15–49 years old occurring in the same period

(continued)

Indicator name	Definition	Numerator	Denominator
Education			
Primary school net enrolment ratio or attendance ratio	Number of children enrolled in or attending primary school who are of official primary school age or higher, expressed as a percentage of the total number of children of official primary school age	Number of children enrolled in or attending primary school who are of official primary school age	Total number of children who are of official primary school age
Gender parity index (primary school)	Ratio of proportion of girls to proportion of boys in primary education	Net primary school enrolment/attendance ratio for girls	Net primary school enrolment/attendance ratio for boys
Water and Sanitation			
Drinking water coverage	Percentage of the population using improved drinking-water source	*Piped into dwelling, plot or yard* – Number of household members living in households using piped drinking-water connection located inside the user's dwelling, plot or yard *Other improved* – Number of household members living in households using public taps or standpipes, tube wells or boreholes, protected dug wells, protected springs or rainwater collection	Total number of household members in households surveyed
	Percentage of the population using unimproved drinking-water source	*Unimproved* – Number of household members living in households using unprotected dug well; unprotected spring cart with small tank/drum; tanker truck; surface water (river dam, lake, pond, stream, canal, irrigation channels); and bottled water	
Sanitation	Percentage of the population using an improved sanitation facility	*Improved* – Number of household members using improved sanitation facilities (facilities that ensure hygienic separation of human excreta from human contact), including flush or pour flush toilet/latrine to piped sewer system, septic tank or pit latrine; ventilated improved pit (VIP) latrine; pit latrine with slab; and composting toilet	Total number of household members in households surveyed
	Percentage of the population using unimproved sanitation facilities	*Shared* – Number of household members using sanitation facilities of an otherwise acceptable type shared between two or more households including public toilets *Unimproved* – Number of household members using sanitation facilities that do not ensure hygienic separation of human excreta from human contact, including pit latrines without a slab or platform, hanging latrines and bucket latrines *Open defecation* – Number of household members defecating in fields, forests, bushes, bodies of water or other open spaces	Total number of household members in households surveyed

DEFINITIONS OF POLICY INDICATORS

Indicator	Indicator definition	Criteria for ranking
International Code of Marketing of Breastmilk Substitutes	National policy adopted on all provisions stipulated in the International Code of Marketing of Breastmilk Substitutes	*Yes*: All provisions of the International Code adopted in legislation *Partial*: Voluntary agreements or some provisions of the International Code adopted in legislation *No*: No legislation and no voluntary agreements adopted in relation to the International Code
Maternity protection in accordance with International Labour Organization (ILO) Convention no. 183	ILO Convention no. 183 ratified by the country	*Yes*: ILO Convention no. 183 ratified *Partial*: ILO Convention no. 183 not ratified but previous maternity convention ratified *No*: No ratification of any maternity protection convention
National guidelines for management of severe acute malnutrition (SAM) incorporating the community-based approach	Indicates the status of each country regarding adoption of national guidelines on management of SAM incorporating the community-based approach	*Yes*: National guidelines have been adopted *Partial*: National guidelines are at some stage of development (e.g., process started, pending finalization) *No*: National guidelines have not been adopted and the process of development has not been initiated *Not applicable*: The country's wasting rate does not merit development of such guidelines (e.g., wasting rate is too low)
New oral rehydration salts (ORS) formula and zinc for management of diarrhoea	National policy guidelines adopted on management of diarrhoea with low osmolarity oral rehydration salts (ORS) and zinc supplements	*Yes*: Low osmolarity ORS and zinc supplements in national policy *Partial*: Low osmolarity ORS or zinc supplements in national policy *No*: Low ORS and zinc supplements not promoted in national policy
Community treatment of pneumonia with antibiotics	National policy adopted authorizing community health workers to identify and manage pneumonia with antibiotics	*Yes*: Community health workers authorized to give antibiotics for pneumonia *Partial*: No national policy but some implementation of community-based management of pneumonia *No*: No national policy and no implementation

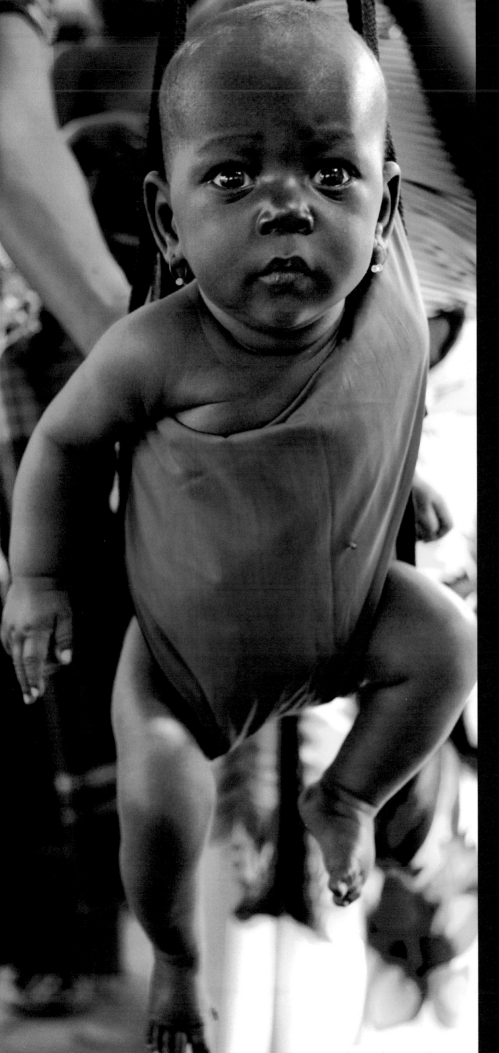

**STATISTICAL
TABLES**

Table 1. Country ranking, based on numbers of moderately and severely stunted children under 5 years old

Ranking	Country	Stunting prevalence (%) 2003–2008	Number of stunted children (thousands) 2008	Percentage of developing world total (195.1 million)
1	India	48	60,788	31.2%
2	China	15	12,685	6.5%
3	Nigeria	41	10,158	5.2%
4	Pakistan	42	9,868	5.1%
5	Indonesia	37	7,688	3.9%
6	Bangladesh	43	7,219	3.7%
7	Ethiopia	51	6,768	3.5%
8	Democratic Republic of the Congo	46	5,382	2.8%
9	Philippines	34	3,617	1.9%
10	United Republic of Tanzania	44	3,359	1.7%
11	Afghanistan	59	2,910	1.5%
12	Egypt	29	2,730	1.4%
13	Viet Nam	36	2,619	1.3%
14	Uganda	38	2,355	1.2%
15	Sudan	40	2,305	1.2%
16	Kenya	35	2,269	1.2%
17	Yemen	58	2,154	1.1%
18	Myanmar	41	1,880	1.0%
19	Nepal	49	1,743	< 1%
20	Mozambique	44	1,670	< 1%
21	Madagascar	53	1,622	< 1%
22	Mexico	16	1,594	< 1%
23	Niger	47	1,473	< 1%
24	South Africa	27	1,425	< 1%
25	Malawi	53	1,368	< 1%
26	Côte d'Ivoire	40	1,246	< 1%
27	Iraq	26	1,175	< 1%
28	Guatemala	54	1,150	< 1%
29	Brazil	7	1,129	< 1%
30	Cameroon	36	1,080	< 1%
31	Burkina Faso	36	1,053	< 1%
32	Zambia	45	1,036	< 1%
33	Russian Federation	13	938	< 1%
34	Ghana	28	929	< 1%
35	Angola	29	926	< 1%
36	Peru	30	886	< 1%
37	Rwanda	51	836	< 1%
38	Mali	38	832	< 1%
39	Chad	41	812	< 1%
40	Syrian Arab Republic	28	778	< 1%
41	Thailand	16	756	< 1%
42	United States of America	3	714	< 1%
43	Democratic People's Republic of Korea	45	704	< 1%
44	Colombia	15	686	< 1%
45	Morocco	23	684	< 1%
46	Cambodia	42	683	< 1%
47	Somalia	42	675	< 1%
48	Turkey	10	674	< 1%
49	Guinea	40	654	< 1%
50	Benin	43	625	< 1%
51	Burundi	53	607	< 1%
52	Zimbabwe	33	570	< 1%
53	Saudi Arabia	20	569	< 1%
54	Algeria	15	496	< 1%
55	Uzbekistan	19	489	< 1%
56	Papua New Guinea	43	405	< 1%
57	Senegal	19	395	< 1%
58	Lao People's Democratic Republic	48	370	< 1%
59	Haiti	29	357	< 1%
60	Eritrea	44	354	< 1%
61	Sierra Leone	36	345	< 1%
62	Venezuela (Bolivarian Republic of)	12	343	< 1%
63	Tajikistan	39	341	< 1%
64	Ecuador	23	323	< 1%
65	Sri Lanka	18	321	< 1%
66	Iran (Islamic Republic of)	5	301	< 1%
67	Honduras	29	282	< 1%
68	Central African Republic	43	280	< 1%
69	Argentina	8	276	< 1%
70	Bolivia (Plurinational State of)	22	271	< 1%
71	Togo	27	255	< 1%
72	Liberia	39	244	< 1%
73	Kazakhstan	17	233	< 1%

(continued)

Ranking	Country	Stunting prevalence (%) 2003–2008	Number of stunted children (thousands) 2008	Percentage of developing world total (195.1 million)
74	Dominican Republic	18	197	< 1%
75	Azerbaijan	25	185	< 1%
76	Congo	30	165	< 1%
77	Mauritania	32	153	< 1%
78	Nicaragua	22	146	< 1%
79	Libyan Arab Jamahiriya	21	145	< 1%
80	Romania	13	136	< 1%
81	Paraguay	18	129	< 1%
82	Guinea-Bissau	47	125	< 1%
83	El Salvador	19	117	< 1%
84	Lesotho	42	113	< 1%
85	Timor-Leste	54	100	< 1%
86	Turkmenistan	19	97	< 1%
87	Kyrgyzstan	18	96	< 1%
88	Jordan	12	90	< 1%
89	Namibia	29	80	< 1%
90	Panama	22	74	< 1%
91	Gambia	28	74	< 1%
92	Occupied Palestinian Territory	10	71	< 1%
93	Botswana	29	64	< 1%
94	Mongolia	27	61	< 1%
95	Kuwait	24	59	< 1%
96	Ukraine	3	58	< 1%
97	Albania	26	57	< 1%
98	United Arab Emirates	17	51	< 1%
99	Tunisia	6	48	< 1%
100	Swaziland	29	46	< 1%
101	Gabon	25	46	< 1%
102	Equatorial Guinea	43	44	< 1%
103	Comoros	44	43	< 1%
104	Montenegro	7	40	< 1%
105	Armenia	18	40	< 1%
106	Oman	13	38	< 1%
107	Uruguay	15	37	< 1%
108	Lebanon	11	35	< 1%
109	Djibouti	33	35	< 1%
110	Bhutan	48	34	< 1%
111	Georgia	13	32	< 1%
112	Cuba	5	31	< 1%
113	Solomon Islands	33	24	< 1%
114	Costa Rica	6	23	< 1%
115	Belarus	4	21	< 1%
116	Republic of Moldova	10	21	< 1%
117	Bosnia and Herzegovina	10	18	< 1%
118	Chile	1	16	< 1%
119	The former Yugoslav Republic of Macedonia	11	12	< 1%
120	Guyana	17	12	< 1%
121	Jamaica	4	9	< 1%
122	Mauritius	10	9	< 1%
123	Singapore	4	9	< 1%
124	Maldives	32	9	< 1%
125	Belize	22	8	< 1%
126	Cape Verde	12	7	< 1%
127	Sao Tome and Principe	29	7	< 1%
128	Bahrain	10	7	< 1%
129	Vanuatu	20	7	< 1%
130	Qatar	8	6	< 1%
131	Suriname	11	5	< 1%
132	Trinidad and Tobago	4	3	< 1%
133	Serbia	7	3	< 1%
134	Croatia	1	2	< 1%
135	Nauru	24	0	< 1%
136	Tuvalu	10	0	< 1%

Note: Estimates are calculated according to the WHO Child Growth Standards, except in cases where data are only available according to the previously used National Center for Health Statistics (NCHS) reference population. Estimates for 96 countries are from surveys conducted in 2003 or later. For more information on countries with estimates calculated according to the NCHS reference population or countries with surveys conducted before 2003, please refer to data notes on page 116.

Table 2. Demographic and nutritional status indicators

Countries and territories	Under-5 mortality rate 2008	Under-5 population (thousands) 2008	% of under-fives (2003–2008*) suffering from: stunting (WHO) moderate & severe	wasting (WHO) moderate & severe	underweight (WHO) moderate & severe	underweight (WHO) severe	underweight (NCHS/WHO) moderate & severe	Average annual rate of reduction of underweight (%) 1990–2008	Progress towards the MDG 1 target	% of infants with low birthweight 2003–2008*
Afghanistan	257	4,907	59 y	9 y	33 y	12 y	39 y	3.1	On track	–
Albania	14	217	26	7	6	2	8	12.7	On track	7
Algeria	41	3,328	15	4	3	1	4	6.1	On track	6
Andorra	4	4	–	–	–	–	–	–	–	–
Angola	220	3,170	29 y	8 y	16 y	7 y	–	7.6	On track	12 x
Antigua and Barbuda	12	4	–	–	–	–	–	–	–	5
Argentina	16	3,361	8 y	1 y	2 y	0 y	4 y	3.5	On track	7
Armenia	23	221	18	5	4	1	4	-2.0	On track	7
Australia	6	1,327	–	–	–	–	–	–	–	7 x
Austria	4	391	–	–	–	–	–	–	–	7 x
Azerbaijan	36	738	25	7	8	2	10	1.6	Insufficient progress	10
Bahamas	13	28	–	–	–	–	–	–	–	11
Bahrain	12	69	10 z	5 z	–	2 z	9 x	–	–	8 x
Bangladesh	54	16,710	43	17	41	12	46	2.3	Insufficient progress	22
Barbados	11	14	–	–	–	–	–	–	–	14
Belarus	13	472	4	2	1	1	1	–	On track	4
Belgium	5	590	–	–	–	–	–	–	–	8 x
Belize	19	36	22	2	4	1	6	-0.2	No progress	7
Benin	121	1,450	43	8	18	5	23	2.2	Insufficient progress	15
Bhutan	81	71	48 x	3 x	14 x	3 x	19 x	6.4	On track	15 x
Bolivia (Plurinational State of)	54	1,245	22 z	1 z	–	1 z	6	3.4	On track	7
Bosnia and Herzegovina	15	172	10	4	1	0	2	18.2	On track	5
Botswana	31	221	29 x	6 x	11 x	4 x	13 x	7.8	On track	10 x
Brazil	22	16,125	7	2	2	–	–	3.0	On track	8
Brunei Darussalam	7	37	–	–	–	–	–	–	–	10 x
Bulgaria	11	349	–	–	–	–	–	–	–	9
Burkina Faso	169	2,934	36 z	19 z	–	–	32	-0.4	No progress	16
Burundi	168	1,155	53 z	7 z	35	14 z	39	-0.2	No progress	11
Cambodia	90	1,611	42	9	28	7	36	4.2	On track	14
Cameroon	131	3,016	36	7	16	5	19	-2.3	No progress	11
Canada	6	1,753	–	–	–	–	–	–	–	6 x
Cape Verde	29	59	12 z	7 z	–	2 z	9 y	3.0	On track	6
Central African Republic	173	656	43	12	24	8	29	-1.6	No progress	13
Chad	209	1,985	41 z	14 z	–	14 z	37	0.7	Insufficient progress	22
Chile	9	1,238	1 z	0 z	–	–	1 y	2.3	On track	6
China	21	86,881	15	–	6	–	7	6.4	On track	4
Colombia	20	4,485	15 y	2 y	5 y	2 y	7 y	2.7	On track	6
Comoros	105	97	44 z	8 z	–	–	25	-3.7	No progress	25 x
Congo	127	551	30	8	11	3	14	2.7	On track	13
Cook Islands	15	2	–	–	–	–	10 x	–	–	3 x
Costa Rica	11	376	6 z	2 z	–	0 z	5 x	–	–	7
Côte d'Ivoire	114	3,139	40	8	16	5	20	1.8	Insufficient progress	17
Croatia	6	208	1 z	1 z	–	–	1 x	–	–	5
Cuba	6	613	5 z	2 z	–	0 z	4	8.5	On track	5
Cyprus	4	49	–	–	–	–	–	–	–	–
Czech Republic	4	519	–	–	–	–	–	–	–	7 x
Democratic People's Republic of Korea	55	1,575	45 y	9 y	18 y	7 y	23 y	–	–	7 x
Democratic Republic of the Congo	199	11,829	46	10	25	8	31	0.8	Insufficient progress	12 x
Denmark	4	320	–	–	–	–	–	–	–	5 x
Djibouti	95	108	33 y	17 y	31 y	9 y	33 y	-2.2	No progress	10
Dominica	11	3	–	–	–	–	–	–	–	10
Dominican Republic	33	1,086	18	3	7	2	4	4.7	On track	11
Ecuador	25	1,392	23 z	2 z	6	1 z	9	2.9	On track	10
Egypt	23	9,447	29	7	6	1	8	2.4	Insufficient progress	13
El Salvador	18	608	19 y	–	6 y	–	9 y	2.7	On track	7
Equatorial Guinea	148	103	43 x	9 x	16 x	5 x	19 x	–	–	13 x
Eritrea	58	811	44 x	15 x	35 x	13 x	40 x	0.7	Insufficient progress	14 x
Estonia	6	73	–	–	–	–	–	–	–	4 x
Ethiopia	109	13,323	51	12	33	11	38	1.7	Insufficient progress	20
Fiji	18	87	–	–	–	–	–	–	–	10
Finland	3	291	–	–	–	–	–	–	–	4 x
France	4	3,870	–	–	–	–	–	–	–	7 x
Gabon	77	182	25 x	4 x	8 x	2 x	12 x	–	–	14 x
Gambia	106	267	28	7	16	4	20	2.1	Insufficient progress	20
Georgia	30	241	13	3	2	1	2	6.3	On track	5
Germany	4	3,446	–	–	–	–	–	–	–	7 x
Ghana	76	3,319	28	9	14	3	–	3.1	On track	9
Greece	4	532	–	–	–	–	–	–	–	8 x
Grenada	15	9	–	–	–	–	–	–	–	9
Guatemala	35	2,118	54 x	2 x	18 x	4 x	23 x	2.7	On track	12 x
Guinea	146	1,635	40	8	21	7	26	0.3	No progress	12

(continued)

Countries and territories	Under-5 mortality rate 2008	Under-5 population (thousands) 2008	stunting (WHO) moderate & severe	wasting (WHO) moderate & severe	underweight (WHO) moderate & severe	underweight (WHO) severe	underweight (NCHS/ WHO) moderate & severe	Average annual rate of reduction of under-weight (%) 1990–2008	Progress towards the MDG 1 target	% of infants with low birthweight 2003–2008*
Guinea-Bissau	195	265	47	8	15	4	19	4.1	On track	24
Guyana	61	69	17	8	10	3	12	2.4	Insufficient progress	19
Haiti	72	1,252	29	10	18	6	22	1.9	Insufficient progress	25
Holy See	–	–	–	–	–	–	–	–		–
Honduras	31	958	29	1	8	1	11	2.8	On track	10
Hungary	7	486	–	–	–	–	–	–		9 x
Iceland	3	22	–	–	–	–	–	–		4 x
India	69	126,642	48	20	43	16	48	0.9	Insufficient progress	28
Indonesia	41	20,891	37	14	18	5	–	2.7	On track	9
Iran (Islamic Republic of)	32	6,402	5 z	4 z	–	–	5	11.6	On track	7
Iraq	44	4,450	26	6	6	2	8	0.6	Insufficient progress	15
Ireland	4	335	–	–	–	–	–	–		6 x
Israel	5	693	–	–	–	–	–	–		8 x
Italy	4	2,892	–	–	–	–	–	–		6 x
Jamaica	31	255	4	2	2	–	–	5.8	On track	12
Japan	4	5,400	–	–	–	–	–	–		8 x
Jordan	20	750	12 x	3 x	4 x	1 x	4 x	4.7	On track	13
Kazakhstan	30	1,384	17	5	4	1	4	0.7	On track	6
Kenya	128	6,540	35 z	6 z	–	4 z	21 y	0.8	Insufficient progress	10
Kiribati	48	10	–	–	–	–	13 x	–		5 x
Kuwait	11	249	24 z	11 z	–	3 z	10 x	–		7 x
Kyrgyzstan	38	547	18	3	2	0	3	12.8	On track	5
Lao People's Democratic Republic	61	776	48	7	31	9	37	1.0	Insufficient progress	11
Latvia	9	109	–	–	–	–	–	–		5 x
Lebanon	13	323	11 z	5 z	–	–	4	-3.3	On track	6 x
Lesotho	79	272	42 y	2 y	14 y	3 y	–	-2.0	No progress	13
Liberia	145	619	39	8	19	6	24	1.5	Insufficient progress	14
Libyan Arab Jamahiriya	17	700	21 x	4 x	4 x	–	5 x	–		7 x
Liechtenstein	2	2	–	–	–	–	–	–		–
Lithuania	7	151	–	–	–	–	–	–		4 x
Luxembourg	3	27	–	–	–	–	–	–		8 x
Madagascar	106	3,060	53	15	36	12	42	-0.4	No progress	17
Malawi	100	2,591	53	4	15	3	21	2.4	Insufficient progress	13
Malaysia	6	2,732	–	–	–	1 z	8	7.6	On track	9 x
Maldives	28	27	32 x	13 x	26 x	7 x	30 x	4.3	On track	22 x
Mali	194	2,207	38	15	27	10	32	1.4	Insufficient progress	19
Malta	6	19	–	–	–	–	–	–		6 x
Marshall Islands	36	6	–	–	–	–	–	–		18
Mauritania	118	475	32 y	12 y	24 y	7 y	31 y	1.5	Insufficient progress	34
Mauritius	17	91	10 z	14 z	–	2 z	15 x	–		14
Mexico	17	10,281	16	2	3	–	5	5.9	On track	8
Micronesia (Federated States of)	39	14	–	–	–	–	15 x	–		18 x
Monaco	4	2	–	–	–	–	–	–		–
Mongolia	41	229	27	3	5	1	6	7.0	On track	6
Montenegro	8	38	7	4	2	1	3	–	On track	4
Morocco	36	3,041	23	10	9	2	10	1.8	Insufficient progress	15
Mozambique	130	3,820	44 z	4 z	–	4 z	18	2.9	On track	15
Myanmar	98	4,629	41	11	30	9	32	1.2	Insufficient progress	15 x
Namibia	42	277	29	8	17	4	21	1.5	Insufficient progress	16
Nauru	45	1	24	1	5	1	–	–		27
Nepal	51	3,535	49	13	39	11	45	0.3	No progress	21
Netherlands	5	958	–	–	–	–	–	–		–
New Zealand	6	288	–	–	–	–	–	–		6 x
Nicaragua	27	675	22	1	6	1	7	4.3	On track	8
Niger	167	3,121	47 y	12 y	36 y	12 y	43 y	0.0	No progress	27
Nigeria	186	25,020	41	14	23	9	27	1.6	Insufficient progress	14
Niue	–	0	–	–	–	–	–	–		0 x
Norway	4	293	–	–	–	–	–	–		5 x
Occupied Palestinian Territory	27	697	10 z	1 z	–	0 z	3	1.3	On track	7
Oman	12	293	13 x	7 x	11 x	2 x	18 x	4.2	On track	9
Pakistan	89	23,778	42 x	14 x	31 x	13 x	38 x	1.7	Insufficient progress	32
Palau	15	2	–	–	–	–	–	–		9 x
Panama	23	345	22 x	1 x	6 x	1 x	8 x	-1.2	No progress	10
Papua New Guinea	69	950	43 y	5 y	18 y	5 y	26 y	–		10
Paraguay	28	736	18	1	3	–	4	-0.1	On track	9
Peru	24	2,975	30	1	6	1	5	3.6	On track	8
Philippines	32	10,701	34	6	21	5	28	0.9	Insufficient progress	20
Poland	7	1,810	–	–	–	–	–	–		6 x
Portugal	4	538	–	–	–	–	–	–		8 x
Qatar	10	77	8 z	2 z	–	–	6 x	–		10 x
Republic of Korea	5	2,292	–	–	–	–	–	–		4 x
Republic of Moldova	17	200	10	5	3	1	4	-3.3	On track	6

Table 2. (continued)

Countries and territories	Under-5 mortality rate 2008	Under-5 population (thousands) 2008	stunting (WHO) moderate & severe	wasting (WHO) moderate & severe	underweight (WHO) moderate & severe	underweight (WHO) severe	underweight (NCHS/WHO) moderate & severe	Average annual rate of reduction of underweight (%) 1990–2008	Progress towards the MDG 1 target	% of infants with low birthweight 2003–2008*
			% of under-fives (2003–2008*) suffering from:							
Romania	14	1,059	13 x	4 x	4 x	1 x	3 x	6.0	On track	8
Russian Federation	13	7,389	13 z	4 z	–	1 z	3 x	–	–	6
Rwanda	112	1,646	51	5	18	4	23	1.9	Insufficient progress	6
Saint Kitts and Nevis	16	2	–	–	–	–	–	–	–	11
Saint Lucia	13	15	–	–	–	–	–	–	–	11
Saint Vincent and the Grenadines	13	9	–	–	–	–	–	–	–	8
Samoa	26	22	–	–	–	–	–	–	–	4 x
San Marino	2	2	–	–	–	–	–	–	–	–
Sao Tome and Principe	98	23	29	9	7	1	9	5.5	On track	8
Saudi Arabia	21	2,859	20 z	11 z	–	3 z	14 x	–	–	11 x
Senegal	108	2,046	19	9	14	4	17	1.1	Insufficient progress	19
Serbia	7	576	7	4	1	0	2	–	On track	5
Seychelles	12	14	–	–	–	–	–	–	–	–
Sierra Leone	194	947	36	10	21	7	–	-0.2	No progress	24
Singapore	3	200	4 x	4 x	3 x	0 x	3 x	–	On track	8 x
Slovakia	8	266	–	–	–	–	–	–	–	7 x
Slovenia	4	94	–	–	–	–	–	–	–	–
Solomon Islands	36	73	33	4	12	2	–	–	–	13
Somalia	200	1,611	42	13	32	12	36	-7.0	No progress	–
South Africa	67	5,200	27 z	5 z	–	3 z	12	-2.6	No progress	15 x
Spain	4	2,373	–	–	–	–	–	–	–	6 x
Sri Lanka	15	1,784	18	15	22	4	–	2.9	On track	18
Sudan	109	5,836	40	16	27	10	31	0.6	Insufficient progress	31 x
Suriname	27	49	11	5	7	1	10	4.8	On track	13 x
Swaziland	83	159	29	3	5	1	7	5.4	On track	9
Sweden	3	527	–	–	–	–	–	–	–	4 x
Switzerland	5	364	–	–	–	–	–	–	–	6 x
Syrian Arab Republic	16	2,807	28	10	9	2	10	2.7	On track	9
Tajikistan	64	871	39	7	15	6	18	–	–	10
Thailand	14	4,843	16	5	7	1	9	5.5	On track	9
The former Yugoslav Republic of Macedonia	11	112	11	3	2	0	2	12.8	On track	6
Timor-Leste	93	185	54 z	25 z	–	15 z	49	-2.3	No progress	12
Togo	98	947	27	6	21	3	21	0.3	No progress	12
Tonga	19	14	–	–	–	–	–	–	–	3 x
Trinidad and Tobago	35	94	4 z	4 z	–	1 z	6 x	1.3	Insufficient progress	19
Tunisia	21	780	6 z	2 z	–	0 z	3	6.6	On track	5
Turkey	22	6,543	10 z	1 z	–	0 z	3	9.2	On track	16 x
Turkmenistan	48	518	19	7	8	2	11	1.7	Insufficient progress	4
Tuvalu	36	1	10	3	2	0	–	–	–	5 x
Uganda	135	6,182	38	6	16	4	20	0.7	Insufficient progress	14
Ukraine	16	2,132	3 z	0 z	–	0 z	1 x	–	On track	4
United Arab Emirates	8	307	17 z	15 z	–	3 z	14 x	–	–	15 x
United Kingdom of Great Britain and Northern Ireland	6	3,601	–	–	–	–	–	–	–	8 x
United Republic of Tanzania	104	7,566	44	4	17	4	22	2.2	Insufficient progress	10
United States of America	8	21,624	3 x	0 x	1 x	0 x	2 x	–	–	8 x
Uruguay	14	249	15 x	2 x	5 x	2 x	5 x	2.2	On track	9
Uzbekistan	38	2,576	19	4	4	1	5	11.4	On track	5
Vanuatu	33	33	20 z	7 z	–	2 z	16	–	–	10
Venezuela (Bolivarian Republic of)	18	2,911	12 z	4 z	–	–	5	1.6	On track	9
Viet Nam	14	7,316	36 z	8 z	–	5 z	20	4.1	On track	7
Yemen	69	3,733	58	15	43	19	46	-3.6	No progress	32 x
Zambia	148	2,282	45	5	15	3	19	1.6	Insufficient progress	11
Zimbabwe	96	1,707	33	7	12	3	17	-1.7	No progress	11

SUMMARY INDICATORS

Africa[a]	132	151,830	40	10	21	7	25	1.0	Insufficient progress	14
Sub-Saharan Africa[s]	144	134,534	42	10	23	8	27	1.1	Insufficient progress	15
Eastern and Southern Africa	120	61,795	45	8	23	7	26	1.3	Insufficient progress	14
West and Central Africa	169	66,795	40	11	22	8	28	1.0	Insufficient progress	16
Middle East and North Africa	43	46,256	32	10	14	5	14	0.8	Insufficient progress	11
Asia	54	323,567	36	17	27	13	31	1.5	Insufficient progress	18
South Asia	76	177,453	48	19	42	15	47	1.2	Insufficient progress	27
East Asia and the Pacific	28	146,114	22	–	11	–	12	3.7	On track	6
Latin America and the Caribbean	23	53,618	14	2	4	–	6	3.3	On track	9
CEE/CIS	23	26,561	–	–	–	–	5	8.8	On track	6
Industrialized countries[t]	6	56,038	–	–	–	–	–	–	–	–
Developing countries[t]	72	566,411	34	13	23	10	26	1.5	Insufficient progress	16
Least developed countries[t]	129	122,674	45	11	28	9	33	1.6	Insufficient progress	17
World	65	634,631	34	13	23	10	26	1.5	Insufficient progress	16

DEFINITIONS OF THE INDICATORS

Under-five mortality rate – Probability of dying between birth and exactly 5 years of age, expressed per 1,000 live births.

Stunting (WHO) – Moderate & severe: Percentage of children 0–59 months old who are below minus two standard deviations from median height for age of the WHO Child Growth Standards.

Wasting (WHO) – Moderate & severe: Percentage of children 0–59 months old who are below minus two standard deviations from median weight for height of the WHO Child Growth Standards.

Underweight (WHO) – Moderate & severe: Percentage of children 0–59 months old who are below minus two standard deviations from median weight for age of WHO Child Growth Standards; **Severe:** Percentage of children 0–59 months old who are below minus three standard deviations from median weight for age of the WHO Child Growth Standards.

Underweight (NCHS/WHO) – Moderate & severe: Percentage of children 0–59 months old who are below minus two standard deviations from median weight for age of the National Center for Health Statistics/World Health Organization (NCHS/WHO) reference population.

Average annual rate of reduction of underweight – Underweight prevalence among children under 5 years old is the indicator used to measure progress towards the MDG target to reduce by half the proportion of people who suffer from hunger. Progress is calculated by comparing the average annual rate of reduction (AARR) based on multiple data estimates available for around the period of 1990–2008 with the AARR needed to achieve a 50 per cent reduction over a 25-year period (1990–2015). The rate of change required to achieve the goal is a constant of 2.8 per cent per year for all countries.

Progress towards the MDG 1 target – Countries and regions are classified according to the following thresholds: **On track:** AARR is 2.6 per cent or more or latest available estimate of underweight prevalence (from 2003 or later) is 5 per cent or less, regardless of AARR. **Insufficient progress:** AARR is between 0.6 per cent and 2.5 per cent, inclusive. **No progress:** AARR is 0.5 per cent or less.

Low birthweight – Percentage of infants weighing less than 2,500 grams at birth.

MAIN DATA SOURCES

Under-five mortality rate – Inter-agency Group for Child Mortality Estimation (IGME), UNICEF, World Health Organization, United Nations Population Division and World Bank.

Under-five population – United Nations Population Division.

Stunting, wasting and underweight – Demographic and Health Surveys (DHS), Multiple Indicator Cluster Surveys (MICS), other national household surveys, UNICEF and WHO.

Low birthweight – DHS, MICS, other national household surveys, data from routine reporting systems, UNICEF.

NOTES

(a) Africa includes sub-Saharan Africa, Algeria, Egypt, the Libyan Arab Jamahiriya, Morocco and Tunisia.

(s) Sub-Saharan Africa includes Djibouti and the Sudan.

(t) Includes territories within each country category or regional group.

– Data not available.

x Data refer to years or periods other than those specified in the column heading, differ from the standard definition or refer to only part of a country. Such data are not included in the calculation of regional and global averages.

y Data refer to years or periods other than those specified in the column heading, differ from the standard definition or refer to only part of a country. Such data are included in the calculation of regional and global averages.

* Data refer to the most recent year available during the period specified in the column heading.

z Estimates according to NCHS/WHO reference population. Refer to underweight moderate and severe (NCHS/WHO) estimate for applicable footnotes. Such data are not included in the calculation of regional and global averages.

For a complete list of countries and territories in the regions and subregions, see page 114.

Table 3. Infant feeding practices and micronutrient indicators

Countries and territories	Annual no. of births (thousands) 2008	Early initiation of breastfeeding (%) 2003–2008	% of children (2003–2008*) who are:			Vitamin A supplementation coverage rate (6–59 months) 2008 full coverage (%)	% of households consuming iodized salt 2003–2008*
			exclusively breastfed (<6 months)	breastfed with complementary food (6–9 months)	still breastfeeding (20–23 months)		
Afghanistan	1,269	–	–	29	54	96	28 y
Albania	46	38	40	69	22	–	60
Algeria	714	50	7	39	22	–	61
Andorra	1	–	–	–	–	–	–
Angola	774	55	11 x	77 x	37 x	82	45
Antigua and Barbuda	1	–	–	–	–	–	–
Argentina	689	–	–	–	28	–	90 x
Armenia	47	28	33	57	15	–	97
Australia	267	–	–	–	–	–	–
Austria	76	–	–	–	–	–	–
Azerbaijan	166	32	12	44	16	90 w	54
Bahamas	6	–	–	–	–	–	–
Bahrain	14	–	34 x	65 x	41 x	–	–
Bangladesh	3,430	43	43	74	91	97	84 y
Barbados	3	–	–	–	–	–	–
Belarus	96	21	9	38	4	–	55 y
Belgium	119	–	–	–	–	–	–
Belize	7	51	10	–	27	–	90 x
Benin	342	54	43	72	57	52	55
Bhutan	15	–	–	–	–	–	96 x
Bolivia (Plurinational State of)	263	61	60	81	40	45	88 y
Bosnia and Herzegovina	34	57	18	29	10	–	62 y
Botswana	47	–	34 x	57 x	11 x	–	66 x
Brazil	3,105	43	40	70	25 y	–	96 y
Brunei Darussalam	8	–	–	–	–	–	–
Bulgaria	73	–	–	–	–	–	100
Burkina Faso	721	20	7	50	85	100	34
Burundi	278	–	45	88	–	80	98 y
Cambodia	361	35	60	82	54	88	73 y
Cameroon	704	20	21	64	21	–	49 y
Canada	353	–	–	–	–	–	–
Cape Verde	12	73	60	80	13	–	0 x
Central African Republic	154	39	23	55	47	68	62
Chad	498	34	2	77	65	0	56
Chile	251	–	–	–	–	–	100 x
China	18,134	–	–	32	15	–	95 y
Colombia	918	49	47	65	32	–	92 y
Comoros	21	25 x	21 x	34 x	45 x	20	82 x
Congo	125	39	19	78	21	10	82
Cook Islands	0	–	19 x	–	–	–	–
Costa Rica	75	–	15	–	49	–	92 x
Côte d'Ivoire	722	25	4	54	37	90	84 y
Croatia	42	–	23 x	–	–	–	90 x
Cuba	118	70	26	47	16	–	88
Cyprus	10	–	–	–	–	–	–
Czech Republic	109	–	–	–	–	–	–
Democratic People's Republic of Korea	327	–	65	31	37	98	40 y
Democratic Republic of the Congo	2,886	48	36	82	64	85	79
Denmark	62	–	–	–	–	–	–
Djibouti	24	55	1	23	18	86	0
Dominica	1	–	–	–	–	–	–
Dominican Republic	224	74	9	62	21	–	19
Ecuador	281	–	40	77	23	–	99 x
Egypt	2,015	56	53	66	35 y	68 w	79
El Salvador	124	33	31	–	–	–	62 x
Equatorial Guinea	25	–	24 x	–	–	–	33 x
Eritrea	182	78 x	52 x	43 x	62 x	49	68 x
Estonia	16	–	–	–	–	–	–
Ethiopia	3,093	69	49	54	88 y	88	20
Fiji	18	57	40	–	–	–	31 x
Finland	59	–	–	–	–	–	–
France	752	–	–	–	–	–	–
Gabon	40	71 x	6 x	62 x	9 x	0	36 x
Gambia	61	48	41	44	53	28	7
Georgia	52	37	11	35	20	–	87
Germany	666	–	–	–	–	–	–
Ghana	757	35	63	75	44	24	32
Greece	107	–	–	–	–	–	–
Grenada	2	–	39 x	–	–	–	–
Guatemala	453	60 x	51 x	67 x	47 x	20	76
Guinea	392	35	48	32	–	94	41
Guinea-Bissau	65	23	16	35	61	66	1

Countries and territories	Annual no. of births (thousands) 2008	Early initiation of breastfeeding (%) 2003–2008	% of children (2003–2008*) who are: exclusively breastfed (<6 months)	breastfed with complementary food (6–9 months)	still breastfeeding (20–23 months)	Vitamin A supplementation coverage rate (6–59 months) 2008 full coverage (%)	% of households consuming iodized salt 2003–2008*
Guyana	14	43	21	34	48	–	–
Haiti	273	44	41	87	35	–	3
Holy See	–	–	–	–	–	–	–
Honduras	202	79	30	69	48	–	80 x
Hungary	99	–	–	–	–	–	–
Iceland	5	–	–	–	–	–	–
India	26,913	25	46	57	77	53	51
Indonesia	4,220	39	32	75	50	86	62 y
Iran (Islamic Republic of)	1,388	56	23	68	58	–	99 y
Iraq	944	31	25	51	36	–	28
Ireland	69	–	–	–	–	–	–
Israel	140	–	–	–	–	–	–
Italy	546	–	–	–	–	–	–
Jamaica	52	62	15	36	24	–	100 x
Japan	1,034	–	–	–	–	–	–
Jordan	157	39	22	66	11	–	88 x
Kazakhstan	304	64	17	39	16	–	92
Kenya	1,506	52	13	84	57	27	91 x
Kiribati	2	–	80 x	–	–	–	–
Kuwait	52	–	12 x	26 x	9 x	–	–
Kyrgyzstan	120	65	32	49	26	99	76
Lao People's Democratic Republic	170	30	26	70	48	–	84 y
Latvia	23	–	–	–	–	–	–
Lebanon	66	–	27 x	35 x	11 x	–	92
Lesotho	59	63	36	79	60	–	91
Liberia	145	67	29	62	47	–	–
Libyan Arab Jamahiriya	147	–	–	–	23 x	–	90 x
Liechtenstein	0	–	–	–	–	–	–
Lithuania	31	–	–	–	–	–	–
Luxembourg	5	–	–	–	–	–	–
Madagascar	687	62	67	78	64	97	75
Malawi	599	58	57	89	72	95	50
Malaysia	551	–	29 x	–	12 x	–	–
Maldives	6	–	10 x	85 x	–	–	44 x
Mali	542	46	38	30	56	97	79
Malta	4	–	–	–	–	–	–
Marshall Islands	1	73	31	77	53	–	–
Mauritania	108	60	16	72	–	87	2
Mauritius	18	–	21 x	–	–	–	0 x
Mexico	2,049	–	38 x	36 x	21 x	–	91
Micronesia (Federated States of)	3	–	60 x	–	–	–	–
Monaco	0	–	–	–	–	–	–
Mongolia	50	78	57	57	65	–	83 y
Montenegro	115	25	19	35	13	–	71 x
Morocco	646	52	31	66	15	–	21
Mozambique	876	63	37	84	54	83	25
Myanmar	1,020	–	15	66	67	94	93
Namibia	59	71	24	72	28	–	63 x
Nauru	0	76	67	65	65 y	–	–
Nepal	732	35	53	75	95	93	63 x
Netherlands	185	–	–	–	–	–	–
New Zealand	58	–	–	–	–	–	83 x
Nicaragua	140	54	31	76	43	–	97
Niger	791	38	4	66	–	92	46
Nigeria	6,028	32	13	75	32	74	97
Niue	0	–	–	–	–	–	–
Norway	58	–	–	–	–	–	–
Occupied Palestinian Territory	148	–	27	–	–	–	86
Oman	61	85 x	–	91 x	73 x	–	69 x
Pakistan	5,337	29	37	36	55	97	17 x
Palau	0	–	59 x	–	–	–	–
Panama	70	–	25 x	38 x	21 x	–	95 x
Papua New Guinea	207	–	56	76	72	–	92
Paraguay	154	21 x	22	60	–	–	94 y
Peru	609	48	69	–	–	–	91
Philippines	2,236	54	34	58	34	86	45
Poland	372	–	–	–	–	–	–
Portugal	105	–	–	–	–	–	–
Qatar	15	–	12 x	48 x	21 x	–	–
Republic of Korea	452	–	–	–	–	–	–
Republic of Moldova	45	65	46	18	2	–	60
Romania	214	–	16	41	–	–	74

Table 3. (continued)

Countries and territories	Annual no. of births (thousands) 2008	Early initiation of breastfeeding (%) 2003–2008	% of children (2003–2008*) who are:			Vitamin A supplementation coverage rate (6–59 months) 2008 full coverage (%)	% of households consuming iodized salt 2003–2008*
			exclusively breastfed (<6 months)	breastfed with complementary food (6–9 months)	still breastfeeding (20–23 months)		
Russian Federation	1,545	–	–	–	–	–	35 y
Rwanda	403	41	88	69	77	–	88
Saint Kitts and Nevis	0	–	56 x	–	–	–	100 x
Saint Lucia	3	–	–	–	–	–	–
Saint Vincent and the Grenadines	2	–	–	–	–	–	–
Samoa	4	–	–	–	–	–	–
San Marino	0	–	–	–	–	–	–
Sao Tome and Principe	5	35	60	60	18	23	37
Saudi Arabia	591	–	31 x	60 x	30 x	–	–
Senegal	470	23	34	61	42	90	41
Serbia	8	17	15	39	8	–	73 x
Seychelles	3	–	–	–	–	–	–
Sierra Leone	223	33	11	73	50	12	45
Singapore	37	–	–	–	–	–	–
Slovakia	55	–	–	–	–	–	–
Slovenia	19	–	–	–	–	–	–
Solomon Islands	16	75	74	81	67	–	–
Somalia	395	26	9	15	35	100	1
South Africa	1,091	61	8	49	31	39	62 x
Spain	491	–	–	–	–	–	–
Sri Lanka	365	–	76	86	83	–	94 y
Sudan	1,296	–	34	56	35	67	11
Suriname	10	34	2	34	15	–	–
Swaziland	35	67	32	77	31	44	80
Sweden	107	–	–	–	–	–	–
Switzerland	73	–	–	–	–	–	–
Syrian Arab Republic	590	32	29	37	16	–	79
Tajikistan	193	61	25	15	34	87	49
Thailand	977	50	5	43	19	–	47
The former Yugoslav Republic of Macedonia	22	–	37 x	8 x	10 x	–	94 y
Timor-Leste	44	–	31	82	35	–	60
Togo	213	53	48	70	–	64	25
Tonga	3	–	62 x	–	–	–	–
Trinidad and Tobago	20	41	13	43	22	–	28
Tunisia	164	87	6	61	15	–	97 x
Turkey	1,348	52 x	40	71	26 y	–	69
Turkmenistan	111	60	11	54	37	–	87
Tuvalu	0	–	35	40	51 y	–	–
Uganda	1,466	42	60	80	54	67	96
Ukraine	459	41	18	55	6	–	18
United Arab Emirates	63	–	34 x	52 x	29 x	–	–
United Kingdom of Great Britain and Northern Ireland	743	–	–	–	–	–	–
United Republic of Tanzania	1,771	67	41	91	55	93	43
United States of America	4,399	–	–	–	–	–	–
Uruguay	50	60	57	35	28	–	–
Uzbekistan	553	67	26	45	38	38	53
Vanuatu	7	72	40	62	32	–	23
Venezuela (Bolivarian Republic of)	599	–	7 x	50 x	31 x	–	90 x
Viet Nam	1,494	58	17	70	23	98 w	93
Yemen	846	30	12	76	–	–	30
Zambia	542	57	61	93	42	96	77 x
Zimbabwe	378	69	22	79	40 y	20	91 y

SUMMARY INDICATORS

Africa[a]	35,318	47	32	69	49	73	60
Sub-Saharan Africa[s]	31,632	46	31	70	52	73	60
Eastern and Southern Africa	14,283	59	42	72	61	73	48
West and Central Africa	16,029	36	22	70	45	73	73
Middle East and North Africa	9,941	47	30	60	34	–	60
Asia	68,409	31 **	41	51	53	70 **	73
South Asia	38,067	27	45	55	75	65	55
East Asia and the Pacific	30,342	46 **	–	45	26	89 **	86
Latin America and the Caribbean	10,768	48	41	69	28	–	89
CEE/CIS	5,593	–	27	53	23	–	51
Industrialized countries[t]	11,218	–	–	–	–	–	–
Developing countries[t]	122,474	39 **	37	58	50	71 **	72
Least developed countries[t]	28,302	49	39	69	67	85	57
World	136,241	39 **	37	57	49	71 **	70

DEFINITIONS OF THE INDICATORS

Early initiation of breastfeeding – Percentage of infants who are put to the breast within one hour of birth.

Exclusively breastfed (<6 months) – Percentage of infants younger than 6 months old who are exclusively breastfed.

Breastfed with complementary food (6–9 months) – Percentage of infants 6–9 months old who are breastfed and receive complementary food.

Still breastfeeding – Percentage of children 20–23 months old who are currently breastfeeding.

Vitamin A supplementation (full coverage) – The estimated percentage of children 6–59 months old reached with two doses of vitamin A supplementation in 2008. Full coverage with vitamin A supplementation is reported as the lower of two annual coverage points, i.e., lower point between round 1 (January–June) and round 2 (July–December) of 2008.

Iodized salt consumption – Percentage of households consuming adequately iodized salt (15 parts per million or more).

MAIN DATA SOURCES

Births – United Nations Population Division.

Breastfeeding – DHS, MICS, other national household surveys and UNICEF.

Vitamin A – UNICEF.

Salt iodization – DHS, MICS, other national household surveys and UNICEF.

NOTES

(a) Africa includes sub-Saharan Africa, Algeria, Egypt, the Libyan Arab Jamahiriya, Morocco and Tunisia.

(s) Sub-Saharan Africa includes Djibouti and the Sudan.

(t) Includes territories within each country category or regional group.

– Data not available.

x Data refer to years or periods other than those specified in the column heading, differ from the standard definition or refer to only part of a country. Such data are not included in the calculation of regional and global averages.

y Data refer to years or periods other than those specified in the column heading, differ from the standard definition or refer to only part of a country. Such data are included in the calculation of regional and global averages.

w Identifies countries with national vitamin A supplementation programmes targeted towards a reduced age range. Coverage figure is reported as targeted.

* Data refer to the most recent year available during the period specified in the column heading.

** Excludes China.

For a complete list of countries and territories in the regions and subregions, see page 114.

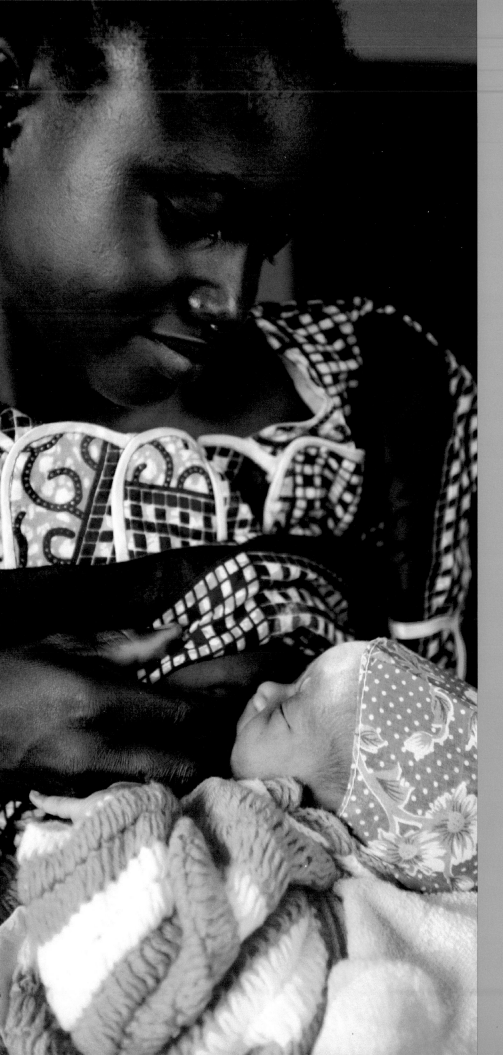

ANNEXES

SUMMARY INDICATORS

Averages presented at the end of Table 2 on page 106 and Table 3 on page 110 are calculated using data from the countries and territories as classified below.

Changes in UNICEF regional and country classifications

In addition to reporting on countries according to its standard regional classifications, UNICEF now reports statistical indicators for Africa and Asia.

Africa includes all countries and territories of Eastern and Southern Africa and of West and Central Africa, as well as the following countries and territories of the Middle East and North Africa: Algeria, Djibouti, Egypt, the Libyan Arab Jamahiriya, Morocco, the Sudan and Tunisia.

Sub-Saharan Africa includes Djibouti and the Sudan, as well as all the countries and territories of Eastern and Southern Africa, and of West and Central Africa. As a consequence of these changes, regional estimates for sub-Saharan Africa appearing in earlier UNICEF publications are not strictly comparable with those published in this report.

Asia includes all countries and territories of South Asia and of East Asia and the Pacific.

Industrialized countries/territories refers to countries and territories that are not included in any of UNICEF's standard regional classifications.

Developing countries/territories are classified as such for purposes of statistical analysis only; there is no convention for classifying countries or territories 'developed' or 'developing' in the United Nations system.

Least developed countries/territories are classified as such by the United Nations.

UNICEF regional classifications

Africa

Sub-Saharan Africa; North Africa (Algeria, Egypt, Libyan Arab Jamahiriya, Morocco, Tunisia)

Sub-Saharan Africa

Eastern and Southern Africa; West and Central Africa; Djibouti and the Sudan

Eastern and Southern Africa

Angola; Botswana; Burundi; Comoros; Eritrea; Ethiopia; Kenya; Lesotho; Madagascar; Malawi; Mauritius; Mozambique; Namibia; Rwanda; Seychelles; Somalia; South Africa; Swaziland; Uganda; United Republic of Tanzania; Zambia; Zimbabwe

West and Central Africa

Benin; Burkina Faso; Cameroon; Cape Verde; Central African Republic; Chad; Congo; Côte d'Ivoire; Democratic Republic of the Congo; Equatorial Guinea; Gabon; Gambia; Ghana; Guinea; Guinea-Bissau; Liberia; Mali; Mauritania; Niger; Nigeria; Sao Tome and Principe; Senegal; Sierra Leone; Togo

Middle East and North Africa

Algeria; Bahrain; Djibouti; Egypt; Iran (Islamic Republic of); Iraq; Jordan; Kuwait; Lebanon; Libyan Arab Jamahiriya; Morocco; Occupied Palestinian Territory; Oman; Qatar; Saudi Arabia; Sudan; Syrian Arab Republic; Tunisia; United Arab Emirates; Yemen

Asia

South Asia; East Asia and the Pacific

South Asia

Afghanistan; Bangladesh; Bhutan; India; Maldives; Nepal; Pakistan; Sri Lanka

East Asia and the Pacific

Brunei Darussalam; Cambodia; China; Cook Islands; Democratic People's Republic of Korea; Fiji; Indonesia; Kiribati; Lao People's Democratic Republic; Malaysia; Marshall Islands; Micronesia (Federated States of); Mongolia; Myanmar; Nauru; Niue; Palau; Papua New Guinea; Philippines; Republic of Korea; Samoa; Singapore; Solomon Islands; Thailand; Timor-Leste; Tonga; Tuvalu; Vanuatu; Viet Nam

Antigua and Barbuda; Argentina; Bahamas; Barbados; Belize; Bolivia (Plurinational State of); Brazil; Chile; Colombia; Costa Rica; Cuba; Dominica; Dominican Republic; Ecuador; El Salvador; Grenada; Guatemala; Guyana; Haiti; Honduras; Jamaica; Mexico; Nicaragua; Panama; Paraguay; Peru; Saint Kitts and Nevis; Saint Lucia; Saint Vincent and the Grenadines; Suriname; Trinidad and Tobago; Uruguay; Venezuela (Bolivarian Republic of)

CEE/CIS

Albania; Armenia; Azerbaijan; Belarus; Bosnia and Herzegovina; Bulgaria; Croatia; Georgia; Kazakhstan; Kyrgyzstan; Montenegro; Republic of Moldova; Romania; Russian Federation; Serbia; Tajikistan; The former Yugoslav Republic of Macedonia; Turkey; Turkmenistan; Ukraine; Uzbekistan

UNICEF country classifications

Industrialized countries/territories

Andorra; Australia; Austria; Belgium; Canada; Cyprus; Czech Republic; Denmark; Estonia; Finland; France; Germany; Greece; Holy See; Hungary; Iceland; Ireland; Israel; Italy; Japan; Latvia; Liechtenstein; Lithuania; Luxembourg; Malta; Monaco; Netherlands; New Zealand; Norway; Poland; Portugal; San Marino; Slovakia; Slovenia; Spain; Sweden; Switzerland; United Kingdom of Great Britain and Northern Ireland; United States of America

Developing countries/territories

Afghanistan; Algeria; Angola; Antigua and Barbuda; Argentina; Armenia; Azerbaijan; Bahamas; Bahrain; Bangladesh; Barbados; Belize; Benin; Bhutan; Bolivia (Plurinational State of); Botswana; Brazil; Brunei Darussalam; Burkina Faso; Burundi; Cambodia; Cameroon; Cape Verde; Central African Republic; Chad; Chile; China; Colombia; Comoros; Congo; Cook Islands; Costa Rica; Côte d'Ivoire; Cuba; Cyprus; Democratic Republic of the Congo; Democratic People's Republic of Korea; Djibouti; Dominica; Dominican Republic; Ecuador; Egypt; El Salvador; Equatorial Guinea; Eritrea; Ethiopia; Fiji; Gabon; Gambia; Georgia; Ghana; Grenada; Guatemala; Guinea; Guinea-Bissau; Guyana; Haiti; Honduras; India; Indonesia; Iran (Islamic Republic of); Iraq; Israel; Jamaica; Jordan; Kazakhstan; Kenya; Kiribati; Kuwait; Kyrgyzstan; Lao People's Democratic Republic; Lebanon; Lesotho; Liberia; Libyan Arab Jamahiriya; Madagascar; Malawi; Malaysia; Maldives; Mali; Marshall Islands; Mauritania; Mauritius; Mexico; Micronesia (Federated States of); Mongolia; Morocco; Mozambique; Myanmar; Namibia; Nauru; Nepal; Nicaragua; Niger; Nigeria; Niue; Occupied Palestinian Territory; Oman; Pakistan; Palau; Panama; Papua New Guinea; Paraguay; Peru; Philippines; Qatar; Republic of Korea; Rwanda; Saint Kitts and Nevis; Saint Lucia; Saint Vincent and the Grenadines; Samoa; Sao Tome and Principe; Saudi Arabia; Senegal; Seychelles; Sierra Leone; Singapore; Solomon Islands; Somalia; South Africa; Sri Lanka; Sudan; Suriname; Swaziland; Syrian Arab Republic; Tajikistan; Thailand; Timor-Leste; Togo; Tonga; Trinidad and Tobago; Tunisia; Turkey; Turkmenistan; Tuvalu; Uganda; United Arab Emirates; United Republic of Tanzania; Uruguay; Uzbekistan; Vanuatu; Venezuela (Bolivarian Republic of); Viet Nam; Yemen; Zambia; Zimbabwe

Least developed countries/territories

Afghanistan; Angola; Bangladesh; Benin; Bhutan; Burkina Faso; Burundi; Cambodia; Central African Republic; Chad; Comoros; Democratic Republic of the Congo; Djibouti; Equatorial Guinea; Eritrea; Ethiopia; Gambia; Guinea; Guinea-Bissau; Haiti; Kiribati; Lao People's Democratic Republic; Lesotho; Liberia; Madagascar; Malawi; Maldives; Mali; Mauritania; Mozambique; Myanmar; Nepal; Niger; Rwanda; Samoa; Sao Tome and Principe; Senegal; Sierra Leone; Solomon Islands; Somalia; Sudan; Timor-Leste; Togo; Tuvalu; Uganda; United Republic of Tanzania; Vanuatu; Yemen; Zambia

GENERAL NOTES ON THE DATA

The data presented in this report are derived from UNICEF global databases, which include only internationally comparable and statistically sound data. In addition, data from the responsible United Nations organization have been used wherever possible. In the absence of such internationally standardized estimates, the profiles draw on other sources, particularly data drawn from nationally representative household surveys such as Multiple Indicator Cluster Surveys (MICS) and Demographic and Health Surveys (DHS). Data presented reflect the latest available estimates as of mid-2009. More detailed information on methodology and the data sources is available at <www.childinfo.org>.

Nutrition indicators

Overview of international reference population

Prevalence of underweight, stunting and wasting among children under 5 years old is estimated by comparing actual measurements to an international standard reference population. In April 2006, the World Health Organization (WHO) released the WHO Child Growth Standards to replace the widely used National Center for Health Statistics (NCHS)/WHO reference population, which was based on a limited sample of children from the United States of America. The new Child Growth Standards are the result of an intensive study project involving more than 8,000 children from Brazil, Ghana, India, Norway, Oman and the United States of America. Overcoming the technical and biological drawbacks of the old reference, the new standards confirm that children born anywhere in the world and given the optimum start in life have the potential to develop to within the same range of height and weight, i.e., differences in children's growth to age 5 are more influenced by nutrition, feeding practices, environment and health care than genetics or ethnicity.

UNICEF is converting its global databases on children's nutritional status towards the WHO Child Growth Standards. It should be noted that due to the differences between the old reference population and the new standards, prevalence estimates of child anthropometry indicators based on these two references are not readily comparable.

Reference population used in this report

To conform to the new international guidelines regarding reference populations, nutritional status indicators are calculated according to the new WHO Child Growth Standards whenever possible. Current global and regional estimates are based only on the WHO Child Growth Standards. To more accurately calculate progress, trends are based on the NCHS reference population to ensure that estimates are based on the maximum number of data points. In addition, to avoid missing data, current estimates at the country level are always presented according to WHO Child Growth Standards, except for the following countries and territories: Bahrain, Bolivia (Plurinational State of), Burkina Faso, Burundi, Cape Verde, Chad, Chile, Comoros, Cook Islands, Costa Rica, Croatia, Cuba, Ecuador, Iran (Islamic Republic of), Kenya, Kiribati, Kuwait, Lebanon, Libyan Arab Jamahiriya, Malaysia, Mauritius, Micronesia (Federated States of), Mozambique, Occupied Palestinian Territory, Qatar, Russian Federation, Saudi Arabia, South Africa, Timor-Leste, Trinidad and Tobago, Tunisia, Turkey, Ukraine, United Arab Emirates, Vanuatu, Venezuela (Bolivarian Republic of) and Viet Nam.

Dates of estimates used in this report

Throughout this report, estimates presented are from 2003 or later unless otherwise specified. In the stunting, wasting and underweight maps that present individual country or territory data, estimates for 96 countries and territories are from surveys conducted in 2003 or later. Estimates for the following countries are derived from data collected before 2003: Bahrain, Bhutan, Botswana, Cook Islands, Costa Rica, Croatia, Equatorial Guinea, Eritrea, Gabon, Guatemala, Jordan, Kiribati, Kuwait, Libyan Arab Jamahiriya, Maldives, Mauritius, Micronesia (Federated States of), Oman, Pakistan, Panama, Qatar, Romania, Russian Federation, Saudi Arabia, Singapore, Trinidad and Tobago, Ukraine, United Arab Emirates, United States of America and Uruguay.

In the exclusive breastfeeding map that presents individual country data, estimates for 108 countries and territories are from surveys conducted in 2003 or later. Estimates for the following countries are derived from data collected before 2003: Angola, Bahrain, Botswana, Comoros, Cook Islands, Croatia, Equatorial Guinea, Eritrea, Gabon, Grenada, Guatemala, Kiribati, Kuwait, Lebanon, Malaysia, Maldives, Mauritius, Mexico, Micronesia (Federated States of), Palau, Panama, Qatar, Saint Kitts and Nevis, Saudi Arabia, The former Yugoslav Republic of Macedonia, Tonga, United Arab Emirates and Venezuela (Bolivarian Republic of).

Calculation of nutritional status burden

Numbers of children who are stunted, underweight or wasted are cited throughout this report. The approach used to calculate these burden numbers is to multiply the prevalence rate for a particular geographical area by the relevant population for the same area. The prevalence rates are generally based on data collected in 2003 or later. The same method was also used to calculate numbers of newborns with low birthweight, numbers of newborns not weighed at birth and numbers of newborns protected against iodine deficiency disorders. The population estimates for children under five and annual number of births come from the United Nations Population Division and refer to the year 2008.

Low birthweight

The low birthweight incidence reported by household surveys in developing countries is often biased because many infants are not weighed at birth and not included in the calculation. Also, for those whose birthweight is measured, the readings are often clustered around multiples of 500 grams. Therefore, a portion of infants noted as weighing exactly 2,500 grams actually weigh less than 2,500 grams. UNICEF reanalysed data from household surveys to adjust for under-reporting and misreporting, using methodology jointly developed by UNICEF and WHO. The adjusted incidence is usually higher than what is reported by the survey.

Vitamin A supplementation

The 'full coverage' indicator is derived from coverage reported for the period from January–June (round 1) and from July–December (round 2). The lower of the two rounds in a given calendar year is reported as the full coverage estimate. This is a proxy for the proportion of children who received two doses of vitamin A in a given year, approximately six months apart.

Iodized salt consumption trend

The household consumption of iodized salt trend data are based on individual year estimates that have different iodization cut-off levels (expressed in parts per million) and therefore may not be comparable. These data provide a general impression of programme evolution.

Anaemia data

Anaemia data come primarily from the WHO global database on anaemia, which is based on data from household surveys, particularly DHS. Data from individual countries or territories may have a numerator or denominator that varies from the definition in the 'General notes on the data', p. 117. For example, data for anaemia among preschool-age children frequently refer to children 6–59 months old but sometimes refer to a different age range, for example, 0–59 months. For more information, refer to <www.who.int/vmnis/anaemia/data/en/index.html> and <www.measuredhs.com>.

Mortality

Child mortality estimates

The child mortality estimates published in this report (infant mortality rate, under-five mortality rate and under-five deaths) are based on the work of the Inter-agency Group for Child Mortality Estimation, which includes UNICEF, WHO, the United Nations Population Division and the World Bank. The group updates these estimates every year, undertaking a detailed review of all newly available data points, and at times, this review results in adjustments to previously reported estimates. The full time series for all countries and territories is published at <www.childinfo.org> and <www.childmortality.org>, the group's website.

Maternal mortality estimates

Maternal mortality estimates are also presented in this report. 'Reported estimates' are those that come directly from a country's national authorities. 'Adjusted estimates', which refer to the year 2005, are based on the work of the Inter-agency Group for Maternal Mortality Estimation.

The process generates estimates for countries with no national data and adjusts available country data to correct for under-reporting and misclassification. (For more information see *Maternal Mortality in 2005* at <www.childinfo.org/maternal_mortality.html>.)

Other indicators

Population below international poverty line of US$1.25 per day (%)

The World Bank recently announced a new poverty line that is based on revised estimates of purchasing power parity (PPP) price levels around the world. The nutrition profiles reflect this updated poverty line, and thus present the proportion of the population living below US$1.25 per day at 2005 prices, adjusted for PPP. The new poverty threshold reflects revisions to PPP exchange rates based on the results of the 2005 International Comparison Program. The revisions reveal that the cost of living is higher across the developing world than previously estimated. More detailed information on the definition, methodology and sources of the data presented is available at <www.worldbank.org>.

Water and sanitation

The drinking water and sanitation coverage estimates were produced by the WHO-UNICEF Joint Monitoring Programme for Water Supply and Sanitation (JMP). They are the official UN estimates for measuring progress towards the MDG drinking water and sanitation targets and use a standard classification of what constitutes coverage. The JMP does not report the findings of the latest nationally representative household survey or census. Instead, it estimates coverage using a linear regression line that is based on coverage data from all available household sample surveys and censuses. Specific country data can be found at <www.childinfo.org> and at <www.wssinfo.org>.

Primary school net enrolment/attendance ratios

The estimates presented are either the primary school net enrolment ratio (derived from administrative data) or the primary school net attendance ratio (derived from household survey data). In general, if both indicators are available, the primary school net enrolment ratio is preferred unless the data for primary school attendance is considered to be of superior quality.